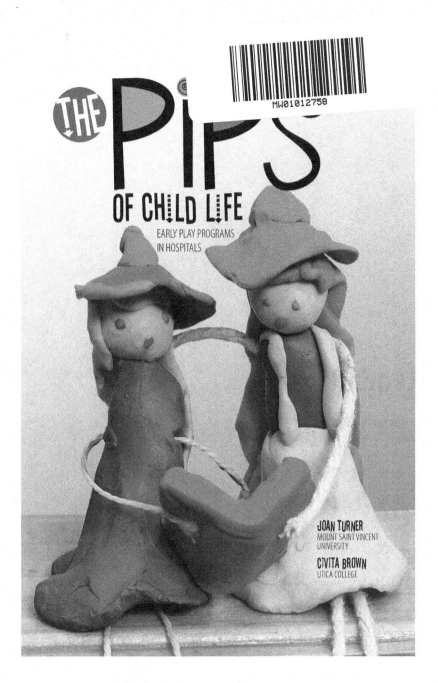

THE PiPs
OF CHiLD LiFE
EARLY PLAY PROGRAMS IN HOSPITALS

JOAN TURNER
MOUNT SAINT VINCENT
UNIVERSITY

CiVITA BROWN
UTICA COLLEGE

Kendall Hunt
publishing company

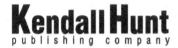

www.kendallhunt.com
Send all inquiries to:
4050 Westmark Drive
Dubuque, IA 52004-1840

Printed in Canada
10 9 8 7 6 5 4 3 2 1

DEDICATION

Thom Brown 1948–2014

Sadly, Dr. Thom Brown passed away at his home in February 2014. I had the pleasure of knowing Thom and note his influence on the development of this text.

When visiting Utica College for the first time I had the honour of meeting Thom in his office. During our casual conversation I learned about Thom's passion for the history of psychology: I remember a set of antique calipers sitting on his desk. It was at this meeting that the real seeds for a history of child life collection were gathered. Through our conversation, an image of how a child life history could be created began to take shape. He generously shared some examples of texts while he talked about his memories of the foundations of the child life academic program at Utica College. He told me his story of Gene Sanford and pondered writing that story to be shared in the future. Of course, he wanted to contribute to our collection.

I am so proud to have placed Thom's composition, *Schools of Thought: The Influence of Theory*, as Chapter One: for that is where it belongs.

—Joan Turner

CONTENTS

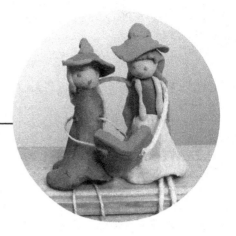

FOREWORD

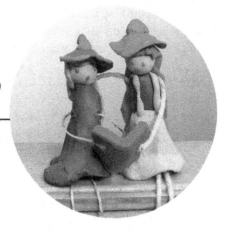

The profession of child life is a relatively young one, and I mean that in two ways. Of the disciplines that typically sit on a healthcare team, physicians, nurses, psychologists, social workers, to name a few, child life is the youngster. While others trace their professional roots back to the 19th century or well beyond, the child life specialist was a 20th-century phenomenon, emerging after medical practice and the care of individuals moved from a home-based setting to the modern

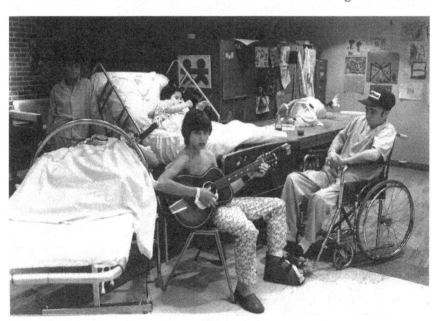

Boys and girl in recreation/play room at Vanderbilt Children's Hospital
Photo courtesy of Eskind Biomedical Library Special Collections

institution of the hospital. The name "child life" itself didn't even appear until midway through the 20th century, and a consensus didn't form around its use as a descriptor of play-based programs in North American hospitals until well after that.

The profession is young enough that many of us who are, shall we say, more senior in the field can trace our professional growth back to a number of the pioneers whose stories are told in the pages of this book. Like other developing professions, people "learned" child life through, in effect, apprenticeships. Coming to the field with a major in early childhood, psychology, child development, or education, the play person got on-the-job training and orientation. Through contacts with our mentors, the oral histories they shared with us, and the occasional conference, we learned what had gone before, how and why the field developed, and which people were instrumental in its origin. In many cases, we were fortunate enough to actually know those pioneers and trace our professional lineage through them to the founding of the profession.

I count myself among this number. When I entered the field at what was then Minneapolis Children's Health Center in what was then the Children's Activity Department, I found that my first supervisor had worked with Mary McLeod Brooks at Philadelphia Children's Hospital. My second supervisor and long-time colleague, Sheila Palm, had been trained in the child life program at Johns Hopkins, introducing me to another set of pioneers, including Jerriann Wilson. The same can be said of many in the field, including the coeditors of this text. Joan Turner was hired at Winnipeg Children's Hospital by Ruth Kettner, one of a number of strong women from Canada who helped form the profession. Civita Brown and I were fortunate enough to have worked with Gene Stanford as he founded the child life program at Utica College. Gene, in turn, had gained his knowledge of child life through a summer program at Wheelock College, where, as he would say, he learned everything he knew from the likes of Muriel Hirt and Evelyn Hausslein. And so it continues...

Now, I recognize that to some readers the names included in the previous paragraph may be just that, names with little other connection or meaning. As I also mentioned, the profession of child life is relatively young. In 2012, a number of us gathered in Washington, D.C., to celebrate the 30th anniversary of the Child Life Council. For many of us in attendance, that span seems like the blink of an eye. Looking around the conference, I realized that that span of time was for others literally a lifetime. As the profession matures, it will become increasingly easy to forget some of its founders and their contributions. The importance of this book, as I see it, is to make sure those memories are not lost, for us to appreciate all that went before. To understand the fortitude that it took for a handful of people, mostly women, to challenge the notions and conventions of the time. To understand what it took to stand up to others and argue that something as messy and uncontrolled as children's play should have a place in the antiseptic healthcare environment. To argue that parents (and eventually, even siblings!) should be present and have a central role in the care of their child. That children should know what is going to happen to them ahead of time and be offered choices and control whenever possible.

Today, we take these things for granted. It almost seems laughable to think that anyone would have objected to their introduction, but these practices were considered radical, even harmful, when first put forward. It took foresight, a compassion for and understanding of the condition of childhood, and most of all courage to bring about this change. For this, we are grateful to those who came before, and to the coeditors and contributors to this book who keep their stories alive.

Richard H. Thompson, Ph.D.
Dean of Arts & Sciences
The College of New Rochelle, New York

 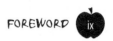

INTRODUCTION

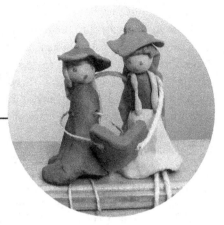

The impact of hospital play and education programs on the healthcare experiences of children and their families can easily be overshadowed by the gift of a well child transitioning home. Even though the play activities experienced by children and their families in today's hospitals far surpass the experiences of earlier generations, families just don't expect play to be a part of their experience. Ask any baby boomer to recall her memories of illness and hospitalization and

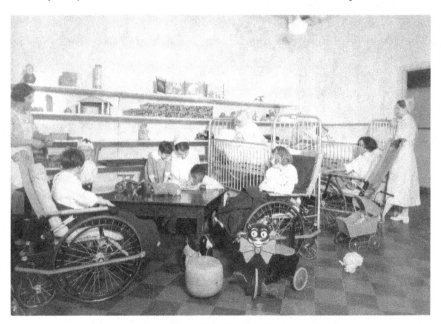

Early activities at The Johns Hopkins Hospital playroom
The Alan Mason Chesney Medical Archives of The Johns Hopkins Medical Institutions

the recollections may be quite dim. For the shift in attitude toward children and play did not translate into programs and services really until the later half of the 20th century, as the baby boomers themselves became parents, now grandparents. Indeed, the early shift began to occur as educated women with an interest and training in child development, early education, and recreation chose to enter the pediatric milieu and create an environment suitable for children. *The Pips of Child Life* offers a glimpse into the early play activities and programs in hospitals and the women who led the way.

Reports of the early days of pediatric healthcare often focus on the medical, technical, scientific, and even architectural advances that have occurred. Yet advances with a unique focus on complementary care and activities for children have also ensued. As the first collection to explore these changes, the contents span the history of play programs starting in the 1900s, a time when pediatrics was just beginning to become accepted as a medical specialty and interest in the well-being of children was advancing—through to the 1970s when B.J. Seabury, Mary Brooks, Emma Plank, and many others promoted the value of play for hospitalized children through interdisciplinary collaborative efforts. In choosing the concept of *pips*, the intention was to reveal the core of play programs relative to the social historical contexts prior to the formation of play as a healthcare profession eventually known as child life.

The title of this history was stimulated by a simple expression that caught my interest:

Long before apples were cultivated it is believed they grew wild.

I sensed the integrity of established child life programs was perhaps taken for granted when our social memory of the past is contracted through a storyline dotted with chronological events. For a deep reflection on the nature of the very early play programs across North America requires greater concentration on the small details scattered across sources and disciplines. To this end, the focus of this collection is the early *pips* found in the Child Life Council Archives at Utica College, in Utica, New York, as enriched through the inclusion of the social historical context of early pediatric hospitalization and play programs. Therefore, each pip from the archive has been chosen for its value as an indicator of the core of activity occurring at any given point in time. It seems these pips and more, scattered far and wide before the establishment of the Child Life Council Archives, are waiting to be gathered and cultivated into stories to be shared.

I first met Civita Brown, both of us certified child life specialists and academicians, at a conference in San Diego, 2008. The spark of connection was Ruth Kettner, early director of the child life program at Winnipeg Children's Hospital and a friend to both of us. Civita and I did not meet again until Boston, 2009, at the Wheelock College Child Life Academic Summit. My interest was peaked when I heard Civita and colleague Lois Pearson mention the ongoing oral history project of the Child Life Council Archives Management Group. We recognized a shared passion for the early days of hospital play and the seeds for a collaborative project were planted. Following two research excursions to Utica College, funded by Mount Saint Vincent University research grants, my interest in the oral history interviews was boosted by those opportunities to literally dig through the contents of the archives. Together, Civita and I agreed if we were going to develop the history of child life for publication, we could not start in the middle of the story, we needed to dig as far back as we could. The result being this first collection: *The Pips of Child Life: Early Play Programs in Hospitals.*

The nine chapters included in this collection were developed as stories composed to share knowledge from the existing records and memories of the early play programs in North America. We did not have to look far for our contributors since those of us with an affinity for the past were already in touch. We are grateful to share the creation of the *Pips of Child Life* with Thom Brown, Leslie Grissim, Lois Pearson, Stefi Rubin, and Jerriann Myers Wilson. Each author offers a unique perspective grounded in their personal association and interest in the history of child life people and programs. We expect readers from a variety of disciplines to appreciate this first look at early hospital play programs and the women who led the way.

A number of individuals have contributed to the progress made in researching and developing the *Pips of Child Life*: Amy E. Caruso Brown, M.D., M.Sc., Marianne Cooney, CCLS, Evelyn Hausslein, MEd., Stephanie Henry, Janine Zabriskie, MEd. CCLS, Lucy Webber, CCLS, Zbigniew Kowalewski, BA (H), and Herb LaGoy (Coordinator of Technical Services & Catalogue Librarian, Utica College). As well, many hospital archivists kindly assisted in the location of documents and photographs for inclusion in the book. Finally, this project would not have been accomplished without the encouragement of the Child Life Council membership.

Joan Turner
Mount Saint Vincent University
Halifax Nova Scotia

 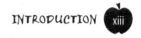

CONTRIBUTING AUTHORS

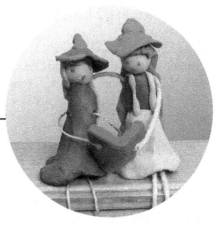

CIVITA BROWN, M.S.ED. CCLS

Civita A. Brown is the Coordinator of Internships for the Psychology–Child Life Department at Utica College and is a CCLS. She has been in the child life and teaching professions for over 30 years. Her research interests include the history of child life and the reduction of stress and anxiety of children prior to surgery. She implemented the CORE/BOCES Child Life Services Program in Oneida County, the first program of its kind in the United States. She also acts as a consultant to area hospitals. Prior to entering academia, she started the first child life program at St. Elizabeth Medical Center and served as Director of Child Life from 1977 to 1981. In addition to teaching, she has given many presentations and workshops on child life issues. She is the author of "The School Setting" in *Child Life Beyond the Hospital*, as well as several articles and abstracts. Her national involvement includes being cochair of the Child Life Council Archives Management Group since 2001.

THOM BROWN, PH.D.

Thomas G. Brown, a former dean and college president, is Distinguished Professor of Psychology at Utica College in Central New York. He has worked and taught there since 1975.Originally from Virginia Beach, he holds a B.A. from the University of Virginia, a M.A. from Hollins University, and a Ph.D. from the University of Maine at Orono. His early scholarship concerned an experimental analysis of animal behavior, but he has increasingly focused on the history of psychology.

LESLIE GRISSIM, M.A., CCLS

Leslie Grissim is a Certified Child Life Specialist at Monroe Carell Jr. Children's Hospital at Vanderbilt. She has been a member of the Child Life Council Archives Management Committee since 1994. Active in the field for over 20 years, Leslie shares her clinical expertise through child life conference presentations and in-services.

LOIS PEARSON, M.ED., CCLS

Lois Pearson is part of the child life faculty in the School of Education at Edgewood College. A Certified Child Life Specialist, she has worked in a variety of clinical settings for more than 30 years. She presently provides child life services to children and families of adult patients in a large adult hospital and trauma center. Lois is the author of chapters in several child life textbooks as well as journal articles. She has cochaired the Child Life Council Archives Management Committee since 2001.

STEFI RUBIN, PH.D.

Stefi Rubin, Ph.D., is an Associate Professor in Child Life and Family Studies at the School of Graduate and Professional Programs, Wheelock College, Boston. A licensed clinical psychologist and family therapist, she is also a clinician at Children's Charter Child and Family Trauma Clinic, Waltham, Massachusetts. From 1996 to 1997, she served on the Board of the Child Life Council. Her research on Emma Plank culminated at the 1995 ACCH Conference where she organized a featured symposium, "The Cleveland Archives Project: The Life and Work of Emma Nuschi Plank," with panelists Marlene Ritchie, Sally Niklas, and Bob Cheshier. In 2005, she contributed to the panel, "Past, Present, and Future: Implications of Emma Plank's Work."

JOAN TURNER, M.SC., PH.D., CCLS

Joan Turner is an Associate Professor in the department of Child and Youth Study at Mount Saint Vincent University, Halifax, Nova Scotia. Joan was the recipient of The Eleanor Blumenthal Fellowship at the University of Missouri–Columbia, Human Development and Family Studies where she graduated with a Doctorate in 2002. She was formerly a Child Life Specialist at Winnipeg's Health Sciences

Centre. A Certified Child Life Specialist, she has been an active member of the Child Life Council including Executive Editor of the Bulletin/Focus publication and member of the Archives Management Committee. Joan authored "Theoretical Foundations of Child Life Practice" in *The Handbook of Child Life* (Thomson, 2009), has published journal articles, and presented at many child life conferences.

JERRIANN MYERS WILSON, M.ED., CCLS

Jerriann Wilson, retired, was the Director of the Child Life Department at Johns Hopkins Children's Center, 1972–2005. She was the first President of the Child Life Council in 1982, and the President of ACCH in 1989. Jerriann received the Child Life Distinguished Service Award in 1992. She has served on a variety of committees within the CLC and currently is participating in the Archives Management Group, the CLC Official Documents Revision Task Force, and the Past Presidents Advisory Group; additional volunteer work includes assisting at the Johns Hopkins Medical Archives in Baltimore.

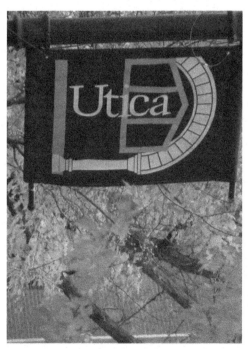

Utica College, Utica New York,
Photo courtesy Zbigniew Kowalewski.
Reprinted with permission.

CHAPTER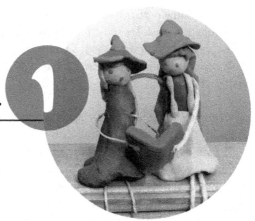

Schools of Thought:
The Influence of Theory

Thom Brown *Utica College*

Nothing happens in a vacuum—not much anyway. There is always a context, and if one wishes to understand why new approaches emerged as they did and when they did, one must evaluate that context.

Ebbinghaus[1] wrote of psychology that it had a long past but only a short history. The same might be said of the child life profession. Its formal history is barely a half century long, but it has roots in a number of different movements that go back considerably earlier. Some of those roots are quite specific, but some are far more general in terms of the breadth of their influence. Among the general elements are intellectual tone, dominant philosophies, social and cultural influences, and so forth that are present in the years leading up to the emergence of play programs and ultimately child life.

Children at the Turn of the Century

During the 1800s, the formal study of children from a psychological standpoint was quite new. The first book devoted specifically to child psychology, Wilhelm T. Preyer's *The Mind of the Child*,[2] wasn't published until 1889. Society's professed attitude toward children (a kind of idealized placement on a pedestal) did not match well with the actual treatment of children, and in some sense, we turned a blind eye toward that reality. Harriet Fraad has noted, "…parents have been other than nurturant in the past and are other than nurturant today. The idea of the nurturant family is a mask for something quite different. Parents in private homes have never been reliable guardians for children. From the beginning of time parents have not only routinely abandoned and neglected their children, but also sexually abused them and battered them."[3]

Attitudes toward children and the way they were treated around the turn of the 20th century depended very much on the social standing of the family. Although it focuses mostly on educational practice, Preyer paints a clear picture of how children were treated relative to their parents' financial status, and it's important to note the differences in treatment between classes.[4] The higher classes have historically treated children better than have those in the lower classes. It appears, though, "that parents have generally treated children as well as their own" situation has permitted.[5]

Children from wealthy families often attended private schools that were basically houses with some rooms dedicated to teaching. With only three or four pupils in each grade, there might be several grades in one room. Girls and boys went to separate gender-specific schools. The public schools were free and attended mostly by children of families with lesser means. They were coeducational, and there was a class of about two dozen for each grade.[6]

The differences in levels of teacher attention could not be more striking, and teachers were harder on children in public schools. If children misbehaved, the teacher might hit them with a paddle or a ruler. Even then, not all children went to the free public schools; many of the poorest were needed to work to help their families financially. Of those who went, most failed to complete the eighth grade and instead worked in factories or farms. Some even became miners.[7,8]

Child labor laws were developed in an attempt to control the worst abuses, and it is at about this time that a juvenile justice system also began to emerge. Courts were to consider first the needs of the child rather than the needs of society. Children were not to be treated as little adults and subject to the same penalties as adults. We find the same issues in the medical treatment of children. Most 19th-century general hospitals occasionally admitted children, and these children were usually placed on adult wards and cared for by a staff with no special training in children's health.

All of these things were about to change.

Historical Antecedents

There was much in the decades before and after the turn of the 20th century that helped form the zeitgeist that ultimately led to improvement in the way children were viewed and treated. On many fronts, concern for "child saving" became the goal. Although there are surely more, at least three developments helped set the stage for all of this: the concept of hospitalism, the influence of psychoanalytic tradition, and the influence of behaviorism.

HOSPITALISM

Hospitalism is a diagnosis originated in the late 1800s and refers to disruptions in the development of language, perceptual and motor skills, and physical maturation arising from hospitalization of infants and children. Depending on where you are on the historical timeline, the cause was generally understood to be lack of social contact when children were isolated in hospitals. In spite of that, at the turn of the century parents were severely restricted from visits to hospitalized children.

Much of the credit for understanding hospitalism has been given to Spitz.[9] He coined the term "anaclitic depression" to refer to the result of such emotional deprivation. When the deprivation lasted longer than five months, however, the problem was more severe, and he called it "hospitalism."

He was not the first to note this condition. Chapin[10] used the term and reported that the earlier the age, the greater the susceptibility. Nor was Chapin the first. Crandall[11] noted that Jacobi, widely considered to be the founder of pediatrics in the United States,[12] used the term "years ago." Crandall wrote:

> Personal care involves much; it is not limited to a bath in the morning, to changing the napkins, and to preparing a bottle at stated intervals. Every child should be taken in the arms when it is fed...frequently turned in their cribs, and kept in proper positions...should receive adequate opportunity for exercise of the limbs. All this requires constant attention. Dr. Chapin is very moderate when he says that one good nurse should be supplied to not more than four or five sick infants, and in some cases one nurse may be required for only two patients. Improper care of infants is far less common in hospitals than inadequate care.

Hospital physicians have not infrequently been blamed by lady managers for what seemed to them improper haste in sending children out of a comfortable hospital ward to an uncomfortable and perhaps unhygienic home. Yet such a course is necessary in most hospitals to save the baby from hospitalism, a disease more deadly than pneumonia or diphtheria.[13]

Although they were not as clear as we are today about the causes of hospitalism, their recommendations for a low nurse-to-patient ratio and the need for return to a home environment as soon as possible suggest an intuitive understanding of the cause.

The clarity that may have been lacking by turn-of-the-century physicians was soon replaced by the work of Spitz,[14,15] and a theoretical basis for this concern would be found in the extensive work of Bowlby,[16] including his brief collaboration with Robertson[17] on mother–child separation and, most recently, his interactions with Ainsworth[18,19] on importance for attachment. It would be wrong to ignore the experiments of Harlow in the 1950s on the devastating effects of maternal deprivation in infant rhesus monkeys,[20] and from 1957 to the mid-1970s Harlow and Bowlby maintained a personal and scientific collaboration.

Beginning with the end of the 19th century, physicians became increasingly concerned about the perils of hospitalization for children although their understanding of the causes remained incomplete. A more robust appreciation of the causal factors and the development of a theoretical framework helped focus the efforts to find solutions that would enhance the psychosocial care given children and adolescents and lead to improved health.

PSYCHOANALYTIC TRADITION

With the most recent turn of the century/millennium, it was popular to generate (and read, of course) top 10 or top 100 lists. When American psychologists were asked to rank the most influential psychologists of the past century, Sigmund Freud was ranked second.[21] B.F. Skinner was first, but the top 10 included Bandura (#3), Piaget (#4), and Erikson (#7), all of who should be identified as theorists of importance for the development of early play programs. That Freud was not first is perhaps surprising given that if you ask almost any layperson to name a psychologist, the name Freud is the one you are most likely to hear. Although much of his theoretical work no longer enjoys widespread acceptance in academic circles, it's difficult to deny the breadth and depth of his influence.

Sigismund Schlomo Freud (1856–1939) wrote extensively, and his collected works fill 24 volumes. His theory, however, is not always internally consistent. It evolved over his career, and at no point did he offer a succinct description of his current thinking. Gaining a good understanding isn't easy, but Hall[22] has carefully summarized the most important elements of the system.

It was Freud's description of the psychosexual stages of development in the child that was the most controversial. He believed that as children progressed through five stages (oral, anal, phallic, latency, genital), they developed habits and proto-types as they resolved the demands of each stage. These, in turn, became elements in each child's personality. The rigors of toilet training and resolution of the Oedi-pus complex were of major importance for one's personality development.[23] When first introduced to a skeptical Victorian Europe, one physician said it sounded like a scientific fairytale.[24] Nevertheless, Freud's system did represent the first of the stage theories of child development that were soon to come. Freud led the way. Among those coming later were Piaget's theory of intellectual development which noted most clearly that children think differently than adults, not just slower[25] and Erikson's theory of psychosocial development with ever-widening circles of interaction,[26] each underpinning therapeutic play practice. In his doctoral disser-tation Kohlberg[27] described stages of moral development, building on the work of Piaget[28] a quarter century earlier, but Kohlberg's theory was less significant for the emergence of therapeutic play than the other stage theories.

Bowlby (1907–1990), Erikson (1902–1994), and Spitz (1887–1974) all identified with the psychoanalytic tradition, but it was Erikson who was the most directly influenced. While teaching in Vienna, Erikson met Anna Freud and even un-derwent psychoanalysis with her. She later trained him in techniques that were centered on child development and psychosexual stages.

Anna Freud (1895–1982) was the youngest child of Sigmund Freud, became a psychoanalyst in her own right, and opened a practice focused on children in 1923. She had begun reading her father's works when she was 15 years old[29] and spent her entire life with him until his death. She did, however, earn international recognition for her work in psychoanalysis in spite of her reliance on her father's theoretical writings for "authority" (Gay, 2006).[30]

Most importantly for this review is her role with the "Matchbox School" in Vi-enna between 1927 and 1932[31] where she applied her psychoanalytic method to childhood education. As she adopted the "progressive child centered approach" that was becoming popular after World War I, she also became a disciple of Maria

Montessori, for obvious reasons. Montessori had lectured in Vienna in 1923,[32] and it was there that Anna Freud learned the details of the Montessori system.

It was also at this school where Erikson taught and became close to Anna Freud. The work and teaching of that trio of Anna Freud, Montessori, and Erikson would have a major influence on our next figure.

Emma Plank (1905–1990) was born in Vienna, and she studied under both Montessori and Anna Freud before immigrating to the United States in 1938 and bringing with her a deep understanding of psychoanalytic theory and technique, especially as applied to children. In a later chapter, her importance in the founding of early play programs in the United States will be described in greater detail as well as the development of the theory and use of therapeutic play.[33]

Beginning in the late 19th century, the evolution of the psychoanalytic tradition under Sigmund Freud ultimately led to the work of Anna Freud, Bowlby, Erikson, Spitz, and ultimately Plank, all of whom helped form that constellation of influences leading to the emergence of the therapeutic use of play.

BEHAVIORISM

Although it may not be the case that behaviorism itself was an important historical antecedent, it's clear the child-related work of its founder, John Broadus Watson (1878–1958), must be acknowledged.

Barely a decade into the 20th century, Watson[34] created a revolution designed to make psychology into the "purely objective experimental branch of natural science" that he believed it ought to be. In doing so, he transformed what psychology was about. He insisted on the rigorous application of the scientific method and wrote that the goals for psychology should include the prediction and control of behavior, a position that ultimately led to the development of behavior modification and therapy. Although they might not have labeled themselves behaviorists—at least in the radical sense that was Watson—both Bandura's social learning theory which stressed the effects of modeling and observation as children learn within a social context[35] and Lazarus's theories about coping with stress[36] were (and remain) behavioral approaches descended directly from Watson's work. Much more recently, the behavioral research of Seligman[37,38,39] (1951, 1991, 1996) on learned helplessness and learned optimism has offered additional theoretical context for practices (like choice and control) that lead to greater resilience.

Watson was a professor and the chairman of psychology at Johns Hopkins University when he conducted his most famous experiment—the Little Albert study—in which he demonstrated that infants could acquire fear and anxiety (over an object or animal) through the standard learning process.[40] They were not built-in reflexes. Although he did not raise the point then, it was surely obvious to those working with children's health that these data strengthened the argument that a child's exposure to environmental pressures (e.g., hospital isolation, parental separation) could lead to the learning of new fears and anxieties and exacerbate existing ones.

Watson should have also eliminated the fear, but he did not—even though one of his graduate students, Mary Cover Jones,[41] had developed behaviorally based techniques to do just that. He was not able to follow through because the university forced him to resign after his messy divorce caused too much embarrassment for the school, which is ironic because he became department chair after his predecessor resigned in similar disgrace.

In *Behaviorism* Watson[42] wrote:

> Give me a dozen healthy infants, well-formed, and my own specified world to bring them up in, and I'll guarantee to take any one at random and train him to become any type of specialist I might select – doctor, lawyer, artist, merchant-chief and, yes, even beggar-man and thief, regardless of his talents, penchants, tendencies, abilities, vocations, and race of his ancestors. I am going beyond my facts and I admit it, but so have the advocates of the contrary, and they have been doing it for many thousands of years.

It is the essence of the radical behaviorism he espoused—all is learned, no behaviors are built-in. Most behaviorally oriented psychologists today would prefer more balance and would insist on some room for genetic influences. The irony for this review, however, can be seen in his *Psychological Care of Infant and Child* (Watson, 1928),[43] a book in which he argued for numerous parenting practices to which most would object today. For example, "treat children with respect but with some emotional detachment." Respect, certainly. Detachment, probably not. Later he recanted and stated he didn't know enough about child development at the time.

Watson's insistence on a more scientific psychology opened the door for later research that led to many more modern theoretical positions; of special note are Rogers, Lazarus, and Seligman. He also helped bring psychology out of the "ivory tower," showing how psychology could develop applications that help everyone in their daily lives.

His psychology was exciting, and it exploded, replacing all the other approaches that were subscribed to in that era. Most importantly, in his work, we find the beginning of the behavioral analysis of child development.

Conclusion

In the second half of the 20th century, play programs were emerging as a practice supported by an existing theoretical base. The roots of that development can be found much earlier though. Historians often write about the zeitgeist, a German term meaning, quite literally, "the spirit of the times," and play has its own particular zeitgeist. Elements within it are (1) a recognition and causal understanding of hospitalism (even in its mildest form), (2) the psychoanalytic tradition, and (3) the revolution that was behaviorism. There can be no doubt that other elements await identification and further study. A more thorough examination of turn-of-the-century societal attitudes toward children and childcare would be a logical next step.

ENDNOTES

1 Hermann Ebbinghaus, *Psychology: An Elementary Textbook*, (Boston: Heath, 1908), 1.
2 William T. Preyer, *The Mind of the Child*, (New York: D. Appleton and Co., 1889).
3 Harriet Fraad, Children as an Exploited Class, *Journal of Psychohistory*, 21, (1993).
4 Preyer, *The Mind of the Child*, 39.
5 Shulasmith Sharar, *Childhood in the Middle Ages*, (London: Routledge, 1990).
6 "American Elementary Schools in the Early 1900s," *OracleThinkQuest*, accessed December 10, 2013, http://library.thinkquest.org/J002606/early1900s.html.
7 Ibid.
8 Marah Gubar, The Victorian Child, *c.*1837-1901, *Representing Childhood* (Pittsburgh: University of Pittsburgh, 2005), http://www.representingchildhood.pitt.edu/victorian.htm.
9 René A. Spitz, Hospitalism—An Inquiry Into the Genesis of Psychiatric Conditions in Early Childhood, *Psychoanalytic Study of the Child*, 1, (1945).
10 Henry D. Chapin, The Babies' Wards of the New York Post-Graduate Hospital, *Archives of Pediatrics*, 14, (1897).
11 Floyd M. Crandall, Hospitalism, *Archives of Pediatrics*, 14, (1897).

12 L.M. Gartner and Abraham Jacobi, *American National Biography*, (New York: Oxford University Press, 1999), 782-784.

13 Crandall, Hospitalism, 448-454.

14 Spitz, Hospitalism, 53-74.

15 René A. Spitz, *The First Year of Life: A Psychoanalytic Study of Normal and Deviant Development of Object Relations*, (New York: International Universities Press, 1965).

16 John Bowlby, Attachment, *Attachment and Loss* (vol. 1, 2nd ed.), (New York: Basic Books, 1965).

17 James Robertson, *A Two Year-Old Goes to Hospital*, (New York: New York University Film Library, 1953).

18 Mary D.S. Ainsworth, Attachment as Related to Mother-Infant Interaction, *Advances in the Study of Behaviour*, 9, (1979).

19 Mary D.S. Ainsworth, Attachments Across the Life Span, *Bulletin of the New York Academy of Medicine*, 61, (1985).

20 Frank C.P. Van der Horst, Helen LeRoy, Helen A., and Réne Van der Veer, When Strangers Meet: John Bowlby and Harry Harlow on Attachment Behavior, *Integrative Psychological and Behavioral Science*, 42, (2008).

21 Steven J. Haggbloom et al. The 100 Most Eminent Psychologists of the 20th Century, *Review of General Psychology*, 6(2), (2002).

22 Calvin Hall, *A Primer of Freudian Psychology*, (New York: New American Library, 1954).

23 Hall, *A Primer of Freudian Psychology*.

24 Peter Gay, *Freud: A Life for Our Time*, (New York: Norton & Co, 2006), 93.

25 Piaget, Jean, *The Moral Judgment of the Child*, (London: Kegan Paul, Trench, Trubner and Co., 1932).

26 Erikson, Erik H, *Childhood and Society*, (New York: W.W. Norton and Co, 1950).

27 Kohlberg, Lawrence, *The Development of Modes of Thinking and Choices in Years 10 to 16*, (Ph. D. Diss, University of Chicago, 1958).

28 Piaget, *The Moral Judgment of the Child*.

29 Gay, *Freud: A Life for Our Time*.

30 Gay, *Freud: A Life for Our Time*.

31 Nick Midgley, The "Matchbox School" (1927-1932): Anna Freud and the Idea of a "Psychoanalytically Informed Education," *Journal of Child Psychotherapy* 3(1), (2008).

32 E.M. Standing, *Maria Montessori: Her Life and Work*, (New York: Plume, 1957).

33 Emma Plank, *Working with Children in Hospitals* (2nd edition), (Cleveland: Press of Case Western Reserve University, 1971).

34 John B. Watson, Psychology as the Behaviorist Views It, *Psychological Review* (1913).

35 Albert Bandura, *Social Learning Theory*, (Englewood Cliffs, NJ: Prentice Hall, 1977).

36 Arnold Lazarus, *Brief but Comprehensive Psychotherapy*, (New York: Springer Publishing Company, 2006).

37 Martin E.P. Seligman, *Helplessness: On Depression, Development, and Death*, (San Francisco: W.H. Freeman, 1975).

38 Martin E.P. Seligman, *Learned Optimism: How to Change Your Mind and Your Life*, (New York: Knopf, 1991).

39 Martin E.P. Seligman, *The Optimistic Child: Proven Program to Safeguard Children from Depression & Build Lifelong Resilience*, (New York: Houghton Mifflin, 1996).
40 John B. Watson and Rosalie Rayner, Conditioned Emotional Reactions, *Journal of Experimental Psychology, 3*, (1920).
41 Mary Cover Jones, A Laboratory Study of Fear: The Case of Peter. *The Pedagogical Seminary, 31*, (1924).
42 John B. Watson, *Behaviorism*, (Chicago: University of Chicago Press, 1930).
43 John B. Watson, *Psychological Care of Infant and Child*, (New York: W. W. Norton & Co., 1928).

BIBLIOGRAPHY

Ainsworth, Mary D.S. Attachment as Related to Mother-Infant Interaction. *Advances in the Study of Behaviour, 9*, (1979): 2-52.
Ainsworth, Mary D.S. Attachments Across the Life Span. *Bulletin of the New York Academy of Medicine, 61*, (1985): 792-812.
"American Elementary Schools in the Early 1900s." *Oracle ThinkQuest*. Accessed December 10, 2013. http://library.thinkquest.org/J002606/early1900s.html.
Bandura, Albert. *Social Learning Theory*. Englewood Cliffs, NJ: Prentice Hall, 1977.
Bowlby, John. Attachment. Attachment and Loss (vol. 1, 2nd ed.). New York: Basic Books, 1965.
Calhoun, Arthur W. *A Social History of the American Family: The Colonial Period* (vol. 1). New York: Barnes and Noble, 1945.
Chapin, Henry D. The Babies' Wards of the New York Post-Graduate Hospital. *Archives of Pediatrics, 14*, (1897): 328-337.
Crandall, Floyd M. Hospitalism. *Archives of Pediatrics, 14*, (1897): 448-454.
Ebbinghaus, Hermann. *Psychology: An Elementary Textbook*. Boston: Heath, 1908.
Erikson, Erik H. Childhood and Society. New York: W.W. Norton and Co, 1950.
Fraad, Harriet. Children as an Exploited Class. *Journal of Psychohistory, 21*, (1993): 37-51.
Gartner, L.M., & Jacobi, Abraham. *American National Biography* (pp. 782-784). New York: Oxford University Press, 1999.
Gay, Peter. *Freud: A Life for Our Time*. New York: Norton & Co, 2006.
Gubar, Marah. The Victorian Child, *c.1837-1901*. *Representing Childhood*. Pittsburgh: University of Pittsburgh, 2005. http://www.representingchildhood.pitt.edu/victorian.htm.
Haggbloom, Steven J., Warnick, Renee, Warnick, Jason E., Jones, Vinessa K., Yarbrough, Gary L., Russell, Tenea M., Borecky, Chris M., McGahhey, Reagan, Powell, John L., Beavers, Jamie, & Monte, Emmanuelle. The 100 Most Eminent Psychologists of the 20th Century. *Review of General Psychology, 6*(2), (2002): 139-152.
Hall, Calvin. *A Primer of Freudian Psychology*. New York: New American Library, 1954.
Jones, Mary Cover. A Laboratory Study of Fear: The Case of Peter. *The Pedagogical Seminary, 31*, (1924): 308-315.
Kohlberg, Lawrence. *The Development of Modes of Thinking and Choices in Years 10 to 16*. Ph. D. Dissertation, University of Chicago, 1958.

Lazarus, Arnold. *Brief but Comprehensive Psychotherapy*. New York: Springer Publishing Company, 2006.

Midgley, Nick. The "Matchbox School" (1927-1932): Anna Freud and the Idea of a "Psychoanalytically Informed Education." *Journal of Child Psychotherapy, 34*(1), (2008): 23-42.

Montessori, Maria. *The Montessori Method*. New York: Frederick A. Stokes Company, 1912.

Piaget, Jean. *The Moral Judgment of the Child*. London: Kegan Paul, Trench, Trubner and Co., 1932.

Plank, Emma. *Working with Children in Hospitals* (2nd ed.). Cleveland: Press of Case Western Reserve University, 1971.

Preyer, William T. *The Mind of the Child*. New York: D. Appleton and Co., 1889.

Robertson, James. *A Two Year-Old Goes to Hospital*. New York: New York University Film Library, 1953.

Seligman, Martin E.P. *Helplessness: On Depression, Development, and Death*. San Francisco: W.H. Freeman, 1975.

Seligman, Martin E.P. *Learned Optimism: How to Change Your Mind and Your Life*. New York: Knopf, 1991.

Seligman, Martin E.P. *The Optimistic Child: Proven Program to Safeguard Children from Depression & Build Lifelong Resilience*. New York: Houghton Mifflin, 1996.

Sharar, Shulasmith. *Childhood in the Middle Ages*. London: Routledge, 1990.

Spitz, René A. Hospitalism—An Inquiry into the Genesis of Psychiatric Conditions in Early Childhood. *Psychoanalytic Study of the Child, 1*, (1945): 53-74.

Spitz, René A. *The First Year of Life: A Psychoanalytic Study of Normal and Deviant Development of Object Relations*. New York: International Universities Press, 1965.

Standing, E.M. *Maria Montessori: Her Life and Work*. New York: Plume, 1957.

Turner, Joan. Theoretical Foundations of Child Life Practice. In *The Handbook of Child Life*, edited by Richard H. Thompson (pp. 23-35). Springfield, IL: C. Thomas, 2011.

Van der Horst, Frank C.P., LeRoy, Helen. A., & Van der Veer, Réne. When Strangers Meet: John Bowlby and Harry Harlow on Attachment Behavior. *Integrative Psychological and Behavioral Science, 42*, (2008): 370-388.

Watson, John B. Psychology as the Behaviorist Views It. *Psychological Review*, (1913): 158–177.

Watson, John B. *Psychological Care of Infant and Child*. New York: W. W. Norton & Co., 1928.

Watson, John B. *Behaviorism* (rev. ed.). Chicago: University of Chicago Press, 1930.

Watson, John B., & Rayner, Rosalie. Conditioned Emotional Reactions. *Journal of Experimental Psychology, 3*, (1920): 1-14.

CHAPTER 2

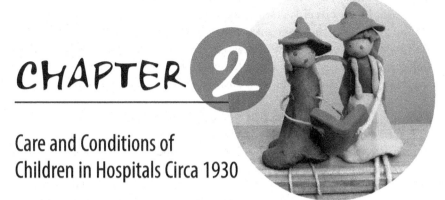

Care and Conditions of Children in Hospitals Circa 1930

Joan Turner *Mount Saint Vincent University*
Leslie Grissim *Monroe Carell Jr. Children's Hospital at Vanderbilt*

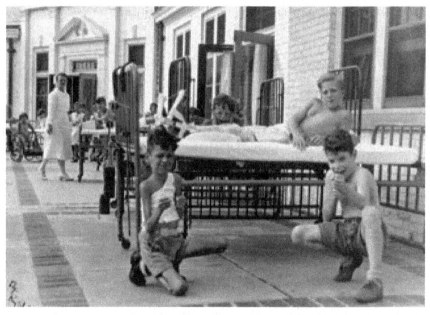

Boys of Milwaukee, Convalescent Home for Children
Reprinted by permission, Children's Hospital of Wisconsin

The imagination is stirred by this photograph of a large group of children posed on the outdoor patio of a children's hospital. Look at the four boys. There's a fifth boy tucked in behind: his fingers waggle, thumb in ear—a comic gesture. The photo originates from Children's Hospital Milwaukee sometime in the 1930s—occasion unknown.[1] Perhaps exposure to the open air and sunlight were a prescribed treatment? Maybe opportunities for outdoor social activity characterized good care? On the other hand, the photo may have been staged for a public relations event. We may never know the answer but we can explore and consider the lives of these children and their stay at the Convalescent Home for Children where they were kept busy with schoolwork, occupational therapy, and other activities.[2]

These boys were growing up during a time of changing attitudes toward children. The White House Conference Children's Charter of 1930[3] represents a marker in time for a shift in attitude toward the health and well-being of children that had been emerging since the turn of the century.[4] Increased urbanization, industrialization, and immigration along with high rates of infant mortality moved the country toward an increasing sentiment for the lives of children. The value of children can be observed through the movements to abolish child labor and introduce kindergarten, playgrounds, and youth clubs. The rise in pediatrics as a specialty and independent children's hospitals was in step with the growth of child experts in a variety of disciplines including nursing, psychology, and early education.

Play Circa 1930s

Growing up during post WWI and the depression era, the boys would have had some exposure to a changing culture of play characterized by an adult intrusion into childhood.[5] Likely city dwellers, the space of their childhood activity, in comparison to rural communities, was constrained by city infrastructure (buildings, roads, businesses), the introduction of the automobile, the creation of playgrounds and sports fields, and a shifting of play activity off the streets and into the backyard. Children on the streets had the potential to come into conflict with adults as play was increasingly relegated into defined spaces, business interests rose in prominence, and cars became faster. As a result, the need to shelter and protect children—to contain and manage their energies—was assigned to experts.

The right of children to play was respected. However, the role of adults in children's play became more pronounced as the science of child development and the promotion of educational play materials and equipment fashioned a level of complexity to play not yet seen. Parallel to the swell of activity around the scientific study of the play life of children was the insertion of trained experts into children's play. For young children, the nursery school was designated as the specialized environment for trained experts to promote appropriate development.[6] At school, knowledge of popular play activities could be used as a strategy to increase relevance in classroom work resulting in genuine interest.[7] On the playground, trained professionals organized activities, promoted "normal" play, and used the "right kind" of materials. However, commercial interests soon became apparent as manufacturers provided outdoor equipment and apparatus for families, playgrounds, and backyards.

In fact, the supervision of play was encouraged as the emerging professionals of psychology and early education cultivated the educational benefits of play. For example, *The Psychology of Play Activities* (1927) compiled "an accurate accounting of what children actually do in their leisure time" and resulted in an "evaluation of the multitudinous activities of childhood in terms of individual or social value."[8] At the time, popular opinion distinguished wholesome and unwholesome play based on the amount of time and energy devoted to the activity, the balance of social participation and alone time, as well as the social contacts involved. However, popular opinion was not a sufficient indicator of value. Therefore, experts trained in "modern" science, development, and education were beginning to become commonplace in those environments frequented by children. The focus on educational play and recreation experts was just beginning and would soon spread to include play programs in hospitals.

By the 1930s, play was so much a part of the American culture that popular toys, books, and other materials were well on their way to being a part of a child's life. Through marketing efforts, movies, cartoons, construction toys, comic books, and games were rolled out as America slowly rose from the depths of the depression: In 1928, Mickey Mouse made his debut in Steamboat Willie.[9] Stacking rings over a pillar as a method to improve infant hand–eye coordination began in the early 1930s.[10] Games such as criss-cross (now Scrabble) and Monopoly and wooden toy bricks called Legos were introduced in the 1930s. Reading materials for entertainment including comic strips (Tarzan, Buck Rogers, Dick Tracy and Flash Gordon) and action comics (Superman and Batman) also made their way into the mainstream starting in the 1930s.[11] The Little Golden Books for younger children were published beginning in 1942.[12] New toys and games—Slinky, Snakes and Ladders, and others—were soon heavily marketed to children and families as the need for play, entertainment, and gifts for celebration or even a hospital stay, became an accepted practice.

Children's Hospitals Circa 1930s

Following the milestone Children's Charter 1930, the American Academy of Pediatrics undertook an extensive survey of leading children's hospitals in North America.[13] Thirty-five children's hospitals in the United States and Canada responded. Study results were reported in the *Journal of Pediatrics* followed by a series of articles (1934–1935) each profiling a major children's hospital or clinic in North America. In his approach to the profile, Dr. Joseph Brennemann, chief of Children's Memorial Hospital Chicago (CMHC), saw the exercise as an opportunity "to portray the personality, the individuality of each clinic or hospital described."[14] Other hospital chiefs used their own unique approach to the task, focusing on the organization and efficiencies of their facility: the end result being a snapshot of the care and conditions of children's hospitals circa 1930s. How fortunate that someone had the foresight to present such a picture. For in combination with the existing literature related to the social and historical context of the period, one can envisage the lives of the boys in the picture both in and outside the hospital.

Many children's hospitals were originally established as charitable institutions funded by endowments with some income from private patients. Over and above the review of the medical campus buildings—their purpose, function, number of beds and disciplines—the series included a glimpse of the services provided in support of the children and families receiving treatment and care. Many, but not all facilities provided convalescent care for long-term acute and chronic patients in addition to outpatient clinics. At the Department of Pediatrics, Johns Hopkins University, the Harriet Lane Home for Invalid Children was established in 1912 and the first pediatric clinic in the United States in 1914.[15] At CMHC, the outpatient departments were growing: the aim was to "keep out, rather than admit, all babies that can be cared for reasonably well or better outside of the wards." [16] As a result, social services workers and volunteers were also required and provided both inpatient and outpatient services to children and families.

In a separate report, "The Committee on Hospitals and Dispensaries: Diet Kitchen, Physiotherapy, X-Ray, Laboratories and Miscellaneous," descriptions of allied services made reference to programs of interest to childcare.[17] According to Smith, 40% of a child's day in the hospital was occupied by medical care; the remaining 60% had the potential to be filled in a constructive way with play.[18] Physiotherapy, occupational therapy, school, and recreation were not yet standard programs in hospitals. Physiotherapy offered facilities for sun treatments—including rooftop solariums and tanks or swimming pools. Southern exposure, open-air wards, porches, windows for light, and ventilation were features for the care of chronically ill children perhaps replicating the benefits of the seaside hospitals of a previous generation.[19] Occupational therapy programs featured activities such as handicrafts and art often assisted by volunteers. School programs were frequently staffed with teachers from the public school system. Records of nursery school and special schools for delinquent boys were also noted. Twenty-two of the 35 responding children's hospitals provided play activities for convalescents. Special teachers and trained playground instructors provided supervision of the play activities, other programs employed "play ladies," "nursery maids," "experienced nurses," or volunteer workers. Some programs were considered well equipped, others haphazard.[20]

The "Nursing" report of that same series focused particularly on the schools of pediatric nurse training.[21] Comprehensive training programs for the care of infants and children were identified at 11 children's hospitals. Of interest here is the following conclusion: "Apparently most of the children's hospitals are not alert to the importance of the training of nurses in normal child psychology and behavior. Comparatively few afford the student nurses experience in kindergarten or nursery school work."[22] Indeed, only one was found to offer an experience in kindergarten work. Interest in the prevention of cross-infection was stated to justify the limitations on bedside visiting and the exchange of toys among patients. Nevertheless, the implementation of play curriculum and training for nurses was soon to advance.

One example, under the guidance of Anne Smith, director of play at CMHC (1932–1937), was the implementation of a play curriculum for nurses training.[23] Bernadine Kern (recreation director) further documented the introductory and advanced course in play at CMHC, in 1939: "Emphasis on play without the use of material equipment has been found to be suitable because it does not require either the time nor labor of getting out and putting away play materials, it can be carried on easily while doing routine nursing care, it enables the student nurses to introduce play even though they may only have a limited time, and it is especially adapted to special precautions and isolation situations."[24] An explicit rejection of the use of commercial materials for hospital play was evident in publications of the time. Examples of types of play were listed by Kern, and include storytelling and story acting, poetry, sign language, tricks, puzzles, nonsense rhymes, tongue twisters, riddles, Mother Goose rhymes, folk songs, nursery songs, song dramatization, finger plays, dramatic play, and games.

The rationale for promoting play without materials was justified due to the fiscal realities of the day and the knowledge of disease transmission prior to the widespread introduction of antibiotics.[25] The toys and books that were available at the time were shared by all the children in the ward and were not specifically selected to meet individual interest or developmental needs. Dolls, teddy bears, rocking horses, blocks, and other common toys were brought into the hospitals by philanthropic families or the families of patients. Indeed, in an effort to combat the introduction of the "unsuitable" play materials, play leaders such as Anne Smith as well as nurses, were also charged with the screening the "gifts" brought in by family members and donors.[26] Educational exchanges with families included information on the suitability of toys; demonstrations and displays of suitable but inexpensive toys, books, and materials; and ideas for the construction of materials at home.

Nurses, and other members of the staff and volunteers, were trained through an interactive method and had supervised experiences on the wards and clinics with the children. Later references to similar training activities of play directors can be noted suggesting this practice was developed in other centers: for example, Susan B. Richards at Mount Zion Hospital, San Francisco late 1930s,[27] and Onica Prall at the Johns Hopkins Children's Hospital around 1943.[28] Further reference to the training of future play leaders across North America can be identified: for example, a Miss Austin trained in Cincinnati and Minneapolis to prepare for her role as the activity supervisor in the new Junior League Activity Department in Winnipeg, 1948.[29]

Hospital Play Programs Circa 1930s

The 1930s were a time in history when women were just beginning to pursue more professional roles in society and wives of professional men began to engage in philanthropic activity. The 19th Amendment, allowing for women's suffrage in the United States, had passed in 1920.[30] Women interested in a career were encouraged into fields such as nursing and education with few entering medicine or academia. Many women of the middle and upper classes chose to volunteer with a variety of activities and special projects sponsored by charitable organizations such as the Junior League and the Kiwanis Club.[31] Although not specifically trained, the volunteers often ran unstructured programs and relied on donations of toys, books, and other materials from community sponsors. Others volunteered and provided play or recreation programs to immigrant children and their families—for example, in settlement houses.

Massachusetts General Hospital is the first program on record to have a trained, non–nurse practitioner to provide play activities for children.[32,33] Miss Isabelle Whittier took on "the unpaid job calling for a trained professional" as the play lady, formally an occupational therapist, for 11 years.[34,35] Dr. Fritz B. Talbot hired the first play lady in 1910; a Miss Hayward, who left her role due to illness. Miss Whittier arrived around 1918 well prepared for the position with previous training in kindergarten and Montessori methods, experience as a library storyteller, and 20 years working with infants at the Boston Settlement Houses.[36] Her description of methods and materials reflected consideration for the age, gender, and nationality of each child in her care. She identified areas where she felt unsuccessful in her role, including difficulties meeting the needs of the oldest boys, procuring a sandbox, and identifying an appropriate substitute for an "unsanitary" live pet that she felt was much needed on the wards. Nevertheless, Dr. Talbot spoke in favor of Miss Whittier: [her work] "has been of more than academic and humanitarian interest because it has been of true therapeutic value and has hastened the cure of the child." [37]

Miss Whittier's retirement from Massachusetts General coincided with extremely difficult economic times throughout the industrialized world. The Roaring Twenties ended abruptly with the stock market crash in October 1929. The Great Depression produced massive numbers of business failures, personal bankruptcies, and unemployment rates exceeding 30%. The poor economic times impacted all of society. Many families could not afford toys; healthcare was fee-for-service and there were no insurance programs, and medical costs were paid out-of-pocket, either in cash or by bartering goods for services; the rates of charity patients increased sharply.[38] Imagine that the boys of Milwaukee were likely from families experiencing similar struggles; therefore, any play-based services provided in the hospital may have been considered an advantage experienced by few children outside the walls of the hospital.

The hospital caregivers for these boys would have been women who were often also charged with leading the play for children in addition to their primary responsibilities. Graduate nurses and student nurses, sisters from religious orders in affiliated hospitals, and volunteers worked together in institutions that were highly structured.[39] The introduction of educated play leaders was just beginning and those leaders were often charged with the training of nurses, student nurses, staff, and members of the community of volunteers in not only play activities, but also the psychology of child development and play.[40,41] Recall the science of childhood was also emerging at this time resulting in the attitude that experts were required to supervise and facilitate the right kind of play. Therefore, although nursing training programs were just beginning to recognize the need for specific curriculum in child development and psychology, some programs were already moving toward the institution of play directors as an essential component of a modern pediatric facility. Early play/education programs have been documented in addition to Massachusetts General Hospital in 1910. The Child Life Council archives at Utica College, in Utica, New York, hold the following records:[42] Mott Children's Hospital in Ann Arbor, Michigan (1922), Babies and Children's Hospital of Columbia Presbyterian, New York (1929), Children's Hospital in Cincinnati (1931), Children's Memorial Hospital in Chicago (1932), and University of Virginia in Charlottesville (1934). Canadian programs include Montreal Children's Hospital in Quebec (1936) and Children's Hospital in Winnipeg, Manitoba (1948).[43]

Early hospital play programs in the 1930s were developed in line with the creation of the U.S. Children's Bureau concerned with the "welfare of children and child life" and the aims of the Children's Charter, White House Conference on Child Health and Protection.[44] Therefore, the start of a movement toward greater attention on the promotion of health, health instruction, wholesome physical activity, and recreation—with teachers and leaders adequately trained—was likely an influence on the experience of these boys at Children's Hospital of Milwaukee. During this period, most inpatient admissions were for prolonged stays; consequently, activity for the convalescing children was a necessity: "To children with fractures who were not really ill, to convalescents nearly ready to be dismissed, to diabetics in the milder stages of the disease, and to many with orthopedic affections, confinement in bed appeared highly irksome imprisonment. In addition to physical limitations, there was sense of being different from other children, a feeling of inferiority, very strong in some, particularly the crippled, the cardiac, and the tuberculosis."[45]

A quote from the 1935 Annual Report, Milwaukee Children's Hospital, provides a good sense of the lives of the boys in the photo: "The Convalescent Home was a wonderful place for those children who are not ready to go back to their own homes. The physical and mental improvements that take place in the child after a short time there are a joy to see. Many of them will carry disabilities for years and some their whole lives, but with the help of our teaching, recreational and curative facilities, good health habits and standards of living are taught which they will take back with them to their homes."[46]

As the demands for hospital care for children increased during this period, so too did the interest in meeting the needs of the whole child as suggested in the Children's Charter.[47] In addition to the separation from family, the prolonged inpatient convalescence also removed a child from formal school programs. As a result, some hospital play programs were educational in focus and often mirrored or were affiliated with school programs in the community. However, as there were no dedicated areas for teaching and play in the early days, the open wards and open-air wards became active areas for playing, teaching, and learning. Perhaps this is the intent behind the photograph of the open-air ward of the Convalescent Home for Children in Milwaukee: to promote the positive side of convalescence for children through an image of group play.

Take another look at the boys in the photo from Children's Hospital Milwaukee. Indeed, the photograph serves as evidence for new attitudes to come: respect for the right for children to play was expanding to the hospital environment and was soon to be embraced as a component of preventive medicine.

ENDNOTES

1 Reprinted with permission: Children's Hospital of Wisconsin.

2 Children's Hospital and Health System, *Children's Hospital of Wisconsin 100 Years of Caring 1894-1994*, (Milwaukee: Children's Hospital of Wisconsin, 1994), 8.

3 The Children's Charter [Government Document], in *Children and Youth in History* (item #124), annotated by Kriste Lindenmeyer, accessed November 21, 2013, https://chnm.gmu.edu/cyh/primary-sources/124.

4 Howard Chudacoff, *Children at Play: An American History*, (New York: NYU Press, 2007), 101.

5 Ibid.

6 Donna Varga, The Historical Ordering of Children's Play as a Developmental Task, *Play and Culture*, 4, (1991): 326.

7 Harvey C. Lehman and Paul A. Witty, *The Psychology of Play Activities*, (New York: A. S. Barnes and Company, 1927), 229.

8 Ibid., iv.

9 Time, *Brief History of Mickey Mouse*, Time Entertainment, http://content.time.com/time/arts/article/0,8599,1859935,00.html .

10 Dr. Toy, *Toy History*, http://www.drtoy.com/toy-history/.

11 Pennsylvania State University, A Chronology of Comic Strips and Comic Books, *Integrative Arts*, 10, http://www.psu.edu/dept/inart10_110/inart10/striptime.html.

12 Random House, *Little Golden Books Timeline*, Random House Kids, http://www.randomhousekids.com/brand/little-golden-books/timeline/ .

13 American Academy of Pediatrics, Report of the Commission on Hospitals and Dispensaries, *Journal of Pediatrics*, 4(3), (1934): 418-425

14 Joseph Brennemann, The Children's Memorial Hospital Chicago, *Journal of Pediatrics*, 4(4), (1934): 523-528.

15 L. Emmett Holt, The Department of Pediatrics Johns Hopkins University, *Journal of Pediatrics*, 4(6), (1934): 811-816.

16 Brennemann, 523.

17 American Academy of Pediatrics, Report of the Committee on Hospitals and Dispensaries (Continued) Diet Kitchen, Physiotherapy, X-ray, Laboratories and Miscellaneous, *Journal of Pediatrics*, 5(2), (1935): 274-278.

18 Anne Smith, *Play for Convalescent Children in Hospital and at Home*, (New York: A.S. Barnes and Company, 1941), ix.

19 Meghan Crnic and Cynthia Connolly, They Can't Help Getting Well Here: Seaside Hospitals for Children in the United States: 1872-1917, *Journal of the History of Childhood and Youth*, 2(2), (2009): 220-233.

20 American Academy of Pediatrics, Report of the Committee on Hospitals and Dispensaries (Continued) Diet Kitchen, Physiotherapy, X-ray, Laboratories and Miscellaneous, 275.

21 American Academy of Pediatrics, Report of the Committee on Hospitals and Dispensaries (Continued) Nursing, *Journal of Pediatrics*, 4(6), (1934): 844.

22 Ibid.

23 Anne Smith, *Report on the Development of Play at Children's Memorial Hospital, Chicago Il*, (Utica, NY: Utica College, Child Life Council Archives, 1937), 14-23.

24 Bernadine Kern, How to Organize a Play Department in the Hospital, *Hospital Management*, (April 1939): np.

25 Clare McCausland, *An Element of Love: A History of the Children's Memorial Hospital of Chicago, Il*, (Chicago: Children's, Memorial Hospital, 1981), chap. 8.

26 Smith, 1937, 9-11.

27 Susan S. Richards and Ernst Wolff, The Organization and Function of Play Activities in the Set-Up of a Pediatric Department: A Report of a Three-Year Experiment," *Mental Hygiene, 24*, (1940): 229-237.

28 J. Alex Haller, The Helen Schnetzer Child Life Program, *The Hospitalized Child and His Family*, eds. J. Alex Haller, James L. Talbert, and Robert H. Dombro, (Baltimore: The Johns Hopkins Press, 1967), 83-85.

29 Children's Hospital Winnipeg, *41st Annual Report Children's Hospital Winnipeg*, (Winnipeg, 1949), 7.

30 Joint Resolution of Congress proposing a constitutional amendment extending the right of suffrage to women, approved June 4, 1919; Ratified Amendments, 1795-1992; General Records of the United States Government Archives. http://www.ourdocuments.gov/doc.php?flash=true&doc=63.

31 See examples in Clare McCausland, *An Element of Love: A History of The Children's Memorial Hospital of Chicago, Il*, (Chicago: The Children's Memorial Hospital, 1981). Anne Smith, *Play for Convalescent Children in Hospital and at Home*, (New York: A.S. Barnes and Company, 1941).

32 Note: Acknowledgment to William E. Russell M.D., Monroe Carrell Jr. Children's Hospital at Vanderbilt for bringing the information to the attention of the Child Life Council Archives Group, November 2013.

33 Note: Massachusetts General Hospital was not included in the American Academy of Pediatrics Report on the Commission on Hospitals and Dispensaries, 1934.

34 Frank Sibley, When Sick People Want Things To Do, *Daily Boston Globe*, (May 19, 1929): A51.

35 Children's Play in Hospitals, *The Playground*, 26, (1923): 488-489. (Author unknown.)
36 Isabelle Whittier, Occupation for Children in Hospital. *The Modern Hospital*, 1(4), (1922): 135.
37 Ibid., 137.
38 Clare McCausland, chap. 8.
39 Paul Starr, *The Social Transformation of American Medicine*, (USA: Basic Books, 1982), 169-170.
40 Anne Smith, *Play for Convalescent Children in Hospital and at Home*, (New York: A.S. Barnes and Company, 1941).
41 Mabel W. Binner, They Play with You Here, *The Modern Hospital*, 44(2), (1935): 54-58.
42 Child Life Council Archives, Utica College, New York.
43 Civita Brown, Lois Pearson, Jerriann Wilson, and Leslie Grissim, From Seeds to Success: Charting the Course of the Child Life Profession, (Paper presented at the 29th Annual Conference on Professional Issues, Chicago IL, May 26-29, 2011).
44 The Children's Charter [Government Document], in *Children and Youth in History* (item #124), annotated by Kriste Lindenmeyer, accessed November 21, 2013, https://chnm.gmu.edu/cyh/primary-sources/124.
45 Anne Smith, The Psychologic Importance of Play in a Children's Hospital, *Archives of Physical Therapy*, (June 1939): 363.
46 Children's Hospital and Health System, 8.
47 The Children's Charter [Government Document], in *Children and Youth in History* (item #124), annotated by Kriste Lindenmeyer, accessed October 3, 2013, https://chnm.gmu.edu/cyh/primary-sources/124.

BIBLIOGRAPHY

American Academy of Pediatrics. Report of the Commission on Hospitals and Dispensaries. *Journal of Pediatrics*, 4(3), (1934): 418-425.
American Academy of Pediatrics. Report of the Committee on Hospitals and Dispensaries (Continued) Nursing. *Journal of Pediatrics*, 4(6), (1934): 838-844.
American Academy of Pediatrics. Report of the Committee on Hospitals and Dispensaries (Continued) Diet Kitchen, Physiotherapy, X-ray, Laboratories and Miscellaneous. *Journal of Pediatrics*, 5(2), (1935): 274-278.
Binner, Mabel W. They Play with You Here. *The Modern Hospital*, 44(2), (1935): 54-58.
Brennemann, Joseph. The Children's Memorial Hospital Chicago. *Journal of Pediatrics*, 4(4), (1934): 523-528.
Brown, Civita, Pearson, Lois, Wilson, Jerriann, & Grissim, Leslie. From Seeds to Success: Charting the Course of the Child Life Profession (Paper presented at the 29th Annual Conference on Professional Issues, Chicago IL, May 26-29, 2011).
Children's Hospital and Health System. *Children's Hospital of Wisconsin 100 Years of Caring1894-1994*. Milwaukee: Children's Hospital of Wisconsin, 1994.
Children's Hospital Winnipeg. *41ˢᵗ Annual Report Children's Hospital Winnipeg*. Winnipeg, 1949.
Chudacoff, Howard. *Children at Play: An American History*. New York: NYU Press, 2007.

Crnic, Meghan, & Connolly, Cynthia. They Can't Help Getting Well Here: Seaside Hospitals for Children in the United States: 1872-1917. *Journal of the History of Childhood and Youth, 2*(2), (2009): 220-233.

Dr. Toy, *Toy History*, http://www.drtoy.com/toy-history/.

Haller, J. Alex. The Helen Schnetzer Child Life Program, in *The Hospitalized Child and His Family* (pp. 80-86), edited by J. Alex Haller, James L. Talbert, and Robert H. Dombro. Baltimore, MD: The Johns Hopkins Press, 1967.

Holt, L. Emmett. The Department of Pediatrics Johns Hopkins University. *Journal of Pediatrics, 4*(6), (1934): 811-816.

Joint Resolution of Congress proposing a constitutional amendment extending the right of suffrage to women, approved June 4, 1919; Ratified Amendments, 1795-1992; General Records of the United States Government Archives. http://www.ourdocuments.gov/doc.php?flash=true&doc=63

Kern, Bernadine. How to Organize a Play Department in the Hospital. *Hospital Management*, (April 1939): np.

Lehman, Harvey C., & Witty, Paul A. *The Psychology of Play Activities.* New York: A. S. Barnes and Company, 1927.

McCausland, Clare. *An Element of Love: A History of The Children's Memorial Hospital of Chicago, Il.* Chicago: The Children's Memorial Hospital, 1981.

n.a., Children's Play in Hospitals. *The Playground, 26,* (1929): 488-489.

Pennsylvania State University. A Chronology of Comic Strips and Comic Books. *Integrative Arts, 10,* http://www.psu.edu/dept/inart10_110/inart10/striptime.html.

Random House, *Little Golden Books Timeline.* Random House Kids. http://www.randomhousekids.com/brand/little-golden-books/timeline/ .

Richards, Susan S., & Wolff, Ernst. The Organization and Function of Play Activities in the Set-Up of a Pediatric Department: A Report of a Three-Year Experiment. *Mental Hygiene, 24,* (1940): 229-237.

Sibley, Frank. When Sick People Want Things To Do. *Daily Boston Globe,* (May 19, 1929): A51.

Smith, Anne. *Report on the Development of Play at Children's Memorial Hospital, Chicago Il.* Utica, NY: Utica College, Child Life Council Archives, 1937.

Smith, Anne. The Psychologic Importance of Play in a Children's Hospital. *Archives of Physical Therapy,* (June 1939): 361-364, 372.

Smith, Anne. *Play for Convalescent Children in Hospital and at Home.* New York: A.S. Barnes and Company, 1941.

Starr, Paul. *The Social Transformation of American Medicine.* USA: Basic Books, 1982.

The Children's Charter [Government Document], in Children and Youth in History (item #124), annotated by Kriste Lindenmeyer. Accessed November 21, 2013. https://chnm.gmu.edu/cyh/primary-sourc es/124.

Time. *Brief History of Mickey Mouse.* Time Entertainment. http://content.time.com/time/arts/article/0,8599,1859935,00.html.

Varga, Donna. The Historical Ordering of Children's Play as a Developmental Task. *Play and Culture, 4,* (1991): 322-333.

Whittier, Isabelle. Occupation for Children in Hospital. *The Modern Hospital, 1*(4), (1922): np.

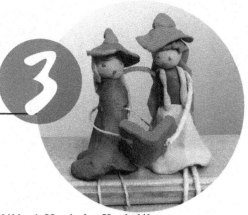

CHAPTER 3

Early Play Programs in Hospitals: 1940s–1970s

Leslie Grissim *Monroe Carell Jr. Children's Hospital at Vanderbilt*
Joan Turner *Mount Saint Vincent University*

Accounts of the early emergence of play programs in hospitals parallel a major shift in the conceptualization of children as the recipients of healthcare. As physicians began to recognize the impact of their care and the condition of hospitals on the emotional well-being of children, policies and programs began to unfold in recognition of the idea that positive changes could be made. By 1940, at least six play programs had been established in the United States and Canada.[1] Although the development of play programs unfolded slowly until the mid-1970s—when about 120 programs are recorded—a closer look at data collected over that period may tell a more complete story.[2] As a new area of care, specialized play programs were showcased as a component of the modern hospital and considered complementary to the advances in medical and technological science of the day.

The Modern Hospital

Two articles published in the *Saturday Evening Post*, in 1947 and 1955, directed the attention of the general reader to the new and modern aspects of hospitals.[3] Photographs of smiling children accompanied by warm and caring doctors, nurses, and volunteers and surrounded by toys, murals, and special visitors illustrated the reporting. The headline, "We're taking better care of children now" summarized the core message: the child was an important focus of care.[4] Early research provided a scientific foundation and raised awareness: "For they knew that real

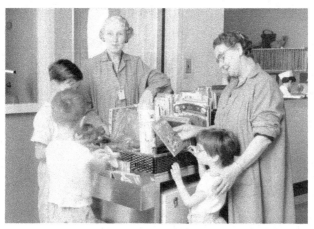

Volunteers and toy cart at
The Children's Hospital of
Winnipeg
WRHA (HSC Archives/Museum)
Series S38-Photographs.
The Children's Hospital of Winni-
peg, reprinted by permission

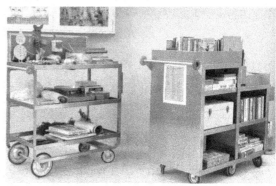

trouble can develop whenever a doctor lets himself think of a child as a small-sized adult."[5] The content of children's books began telling similar stories with books like *Nurse Nancy* (1952) and *Dr. Dan the Bandage Man* (1951) promoting the theme that healthcare is essential to a child's life.[6] The rise of pediatrics, the modernization of children's hospitals, and the increasing birth rate signaled the need for greater attention to children—a need that was soon to be realized.

At the end of WWII, the landscape of North American hospitals began to change. In the United States, the 1946 Hospital Survey and Construction Act provided funds for new construction with the requirement of a provision for free services to the poor.[7] Hospitals were expected to serve all children regardless of race, color, or creed. Carefully considered architecture and design, in addition to the many hospital "specialties"—including play programs—were becoming essential features that evoked great pride in the United States and Canada. *The Canadian Hospital* featured an example of a modern children's hospital in October 1957.[8] The new Winnipeg Children's Hospital, built to replace the original 1911 structure, was financed through community donations in partnership with provincial and federal grants. The article contained a series of feature essays (describing the history, layout, nursing, outpatients, surgery, records, therapies, dietetics, and laboratories) complemented by floor plans and photographs, including the play deck, playroom, and other play areas located throughout the new facility. Attention to the impact of design on emotional well-being was explicit and included a description of the relationship between color choices and patterns and the needs of children, hospital staff, and visitors. Consideration of the perceptions of young children was likewise deliberate: "In order to reduce the corridors to more child-like proportions, the panels under the windows between corridor and wards were painted a series of six intense colours, giving the corridor the appearance of an aisle between rows of toy building blocks."[9] The superintendent expressed their pride, stating, "It is a hospital with a modest past but an unlimited future in which it intends to take its place along with the great pediatric institutions of America."[10]

Respect for children was clearly increasing in importance on many levels. With the establishment of pediatrics as a separate specialty came the formation of numerous child-focused subspecialties and allied health professions. Children's hospitals were composed of a tapestry of care providers all integral to the provision of quality healthcare services. The progress of children's facilities beyond this point in time was intertwined with research and the establishment of research foundations. As physicians became aware of the impact of illness and hospitalization on the progress of their small patients, the care of the whole child finally came into focus.

Early Research on Hospital Play

The work of Bakwin,[11] Spitz,[12] and Prugh[13] progressively legitimized greater attention to the day-to-day activities of the child in hospital—really, attention to the child's life. Documentation by Spitz regarding the influence of the hospital environment on infants, particularly the absence of mothers and stimulation, and Bakwin's recognition of infection prevention policy and practices as harmful to children, advanced the humanization of care. Wojtasik and White have suggested that hospitals were inclined to support the inclusion of volunteers and play programs, rather than parents, as a method to support the needs of children[14]; this practice is reflected in early studies of play for hospitalized children. In fact, Bakwin's wife and colleague, Dr. Ruth Bakwin, a member of the advisory committee for the American Toy Institute's research division, allowed two observational studies of children's interactions with toys at the New York Infirmary in 1948 and 1950 when she was the director of pediatrics.

Langdon[15] and Gips,[16] both associated with Columbia University, conducted exploratory investigations within the natural conditions of a busy hospital. The hospital ward structure grouped the patients by disease (cardiac; general medicine; ear, nose, and throat; and tuberculosis care). Wards consisted of a large room with cribs or beds lined up next to one another. The play space was located in the center of the room, trays were provided for children confined to bed, while mobile children had access to an additional play corner. Both authors acknowledged the limitations of the conditions and the impact of illness and hospitalization on the well-being of children. Given the limited number of nursing staff and restricted visiting hours for parents, an occupational therapist provided most of the play interaction with the toys. The researcher supplied the toys.

The common aim of both studies was to discover the potential value of toys for children in hospital and to suggest ways in which improved design and manufacture of toys could contribute to hospital care. Observational data were collected for each toy as multiple children with varying conditions and needs used it over time. The Langdon study published only summary statements based on observations but the methodology used by Gips provided data on the frequency and duration of use relative to the age of the child for 20 specific toys.

Langdon reported eight main findings, particularly emphasizing the concept of "revealment and expression of feelings."[17] Toys were recognized for their value to the child during critical moments (e.g., admissions, departure of a parent), supporting routines such as naps and bedtime, relieving boredom, increasing morale, preventing problem behavior, and treating physical impairment (e.g., encouraging speech through the use of a toy telephone). As the researchers were not privy to the confidential records of the children, the observations related to the meaning of the children's play were speculative. Children's play with miniatures (dolls, furniture, toys) sometimes suggested family histories of violence, separation, house fires, and evictions. Children used toy telephones to call family: "Sometimes, a child called up his mother and asked her to hurry and come for him."[18] In waiting room play areas, observers documented the comments of the mothers, who were often surprised to see the skills of their child or to recognize themselves in the child's play: "Sounds just like me when I scold the kids."[19] Langdon concluded that toys served a useful and constructive service and should be standard equipment in the hospital.[20]

In the second study, Gips documented findings specific to observations in six categories of toys.[21] Balloons were popular and were viewed as valuable across age groups to motivate physical activity, imagination, or diversion. Pull toys were of interest to mobile children under the age of 5 years. Realistic toys—pony cart, wagons, dogs with a wagging tail, for example—were stated to be preferred over fantasy figures, such as movie characters. Imaginative play was facilitated using nurse and doctor kits, doll families, and train sets. Hospital play was documented: "[A]lmost invariably the 'patient' was so uncooperative to play medication and examination that three 'nurses' had to hold him down, even though these same children almost always were cooperative to actual medication."[22] Additionally, children were noted to reverse roles, with doctors and nurses receiving the treatments. Gips speculated that the imaginary play allowed children to express feelings of fear, loneliness, and anxiety as well as feelings around hospitalization, treatment, and surgery.

Construction toys and manipulative toys were of mixed value.[23] The boys often monopolized the construction toys. Larger blocks encouraged group play over longer periods of time and required some supervision. They were also too heavy for bed play. Gips appreciated the value of invention and constructive activity. In contrast, some manipulative toys held little interest for the children except for brief periods of time. After the action of the toy was observed, the children looked for another activity. Puzzles also did not hold children's interest, although younger children engaged for long periods with lacing and peg hammer toys. Observations of crib toys were very limited with distraction and some exercise noted as benefits.

Gips reached similar conclusions to Langdon and also included suggestions for the care and storage of toys, importance of supervised play, and value of toys for promoting cooperation with care. She also directed attention to the child's expression of emotions, particularly around medical themes. Gips suggested that investigating the value of group play for adjustment to and recovery from illness and hospitalization could be a rewarding avenue of inquiry. Missing from both studies however, was a commitment to the possibility of engaging specific play staff with children or any mention of the benefits of parental involvement. Both Langdon and Gips thought that nurses were sufficient to provide play to promote the adjustment and recovery of children.[24]

Enter the Play Supervisor

Qualified play supervisors on pediatric units were introduced to manage the play opportunities for children. A 1954 report from the Committee on Hospitals and Dispensaries of the American Academy of Pediatrics (AAP) stated, "Every pediatric unit should have recreational space for children to enjoy group play."[25]

Although lay volunteers were common, the shift toward the hiring of a qualified play supervisor, often a teacher, for a salaried position was beginning. In Washington Freedmen's Hospital, a grant-funded part-time position in 1954 became a full-time play supervisor in the regular budget.[26] According to play lady Burma Whitted, "[T]he role of the play supervisor is to extend emotional hospitality, love and affection to a troubled and confused child and to provide suitable entertainment for the well-adjusted youngster in order to maintain a sense of security and well-being."[27] Later descriptions of play programs would directly speak to additional functions whereby the emotional needs of the hospitalized child were addressed. For example, in a 1962 journal article, Blumgart and Korsch reported the play therapist's role in observation and assessment of the child, parental support, exploration of the child's reactions to illness and medical care, and support during medical procedures at The New York Hospital Cornell Medical Center.[28]

The shift toward the integration of play services was clarified in the description of the play program at Boston Floating Hospital from 1956.[29] Operating under the service of the Child Psychiatric Unit, the play teachers were part of the mental health team, and consequently were able to communicate a sense of an advancing program of care for the whole child. Play teachers were located in a central playroom and provided a program described as "similar to that of a nursery school."[30] Play services began early in the day with play teachers, dressed in smocks, visiting the wards to consult with medical staff, deliver play materials, and personally invite those children with medical clearance to visit the playroom. Children changed into play clothes upon arrival and could stay for lunch, returning to the ward for visiting hours between 2 and 3 o'clock. The playroom closed for the day at 4 o'clock, although volunteers were present on the wards during the evening.

Of interest to the theme of advancing play programs is a distinct change in the language used to describe the play program, the experience of the child, and the stated outcomes of the services. For example, when describing the invitation to attend the play program, Tisza and Angoff discussed the implications of providing choices, respecting a child's decision, and the implicit underlying mechanisms of the child's behavior.[31] They pointed to the child's experience and emotional state, individual needs and wants, attitude, abilities and interests, as each influenced the child's response. For example, Tisza and Angoff stated:

> Some children need to be persuaded. They have to be reassured repeatedly that they are really wanted by the teacher. Other children, and this occurs again and again especially with the four to six year olds, remain firm in their refusal. The teacher understands that they have a need to assert themselves success-

fully and accepts the temporary refusal while expressing the hope that they may change their minds later. It is our experience that once the teacher's tolerant attitude gives satisfaction to the child's desire for autonomy the child will become a willing participant in the playgroup - sometimes not later than the afternoon of that same day.[32]

The nondirective technique promoted a permissive and accepting environment for children to play freely. Play teachers emphasized the benefits of freedom and activity that allowed children to maintain their interests and their identity as well as gain mastery as they faced new challenges. Children were free to choose their activities in the playroom and become active agents within an atmosphere of acceptance. Teachers documented their observations, particularly when children had difficulty accepting their illness or adjusting to the hospital. For patients under the care of the psychiatrist, the playroom notes were included as a part of the comprehensive medical study. As members of the mental healthcare team, teachers were in contact with the psychiatrist who visited the playroom daily and supervised the teacher-in-charge. However, not all play programs existed under the umbrella of mental health. As Dombro reported in 1967, programs across the United States and Canada within children's hospitals and within pediatric units of general hospitals were at varying stages of development.[33,34]

Growth of Play Programs

The acceptance of play programs as a component of comprehensive pediatric care was beginning to become noticeable. The concept of integrating play opportunities and play programs requiring trained personnel into the hospital services slowly began to spread during the 1960s, somewhat parallel to the introduction of hospital school programs. Surveys of play programs in the United States and Canada were initiated in the late 1960s, and soon demonstrated the divergence of program approaches and services.

In 1967, Dombro, of the Johns Hopkins Children's Hospital, led two survey initiatives: one for children's hospitals in the United States and Canada and the other for pediatric units within general hospitals. Interested in establishing the state of the development of play programs, Dombro introduced the term "child life" and defined child life programs as those with "staff actively engaged in meeting growth and developmental needs of children."[35] Of 132 surveys sent to children's hospitals, 69% (91) of the questionnaires were returned. Programs were identified in 76% (69)

of the hospitals. Of the 24% (22) who stated the growth and developmental needs of children were provided by nurses, 13 declared they had no need for a separate program but 9 indicated they were interested in starting a program.[36] Over half of the hospitals reported recreational services; however, the staff-to-patient ratio was large and ranged from 1:40 to 1:100 children. In line with the 1954 APA recommendation, almost 60% had specific space for the programs, and some had multiple spaces (e.g., playrooms, schoolrooms, gymnasiums, outdoor playgrounds). Trained staff with higher education (bachelor's or master's degree) were employed in just over a quarter of the programs. The pattern was similar for pediatric units in general hospitals.[37] Of the 36% (151) of the general hospitals that responded to the survey, 61% (92) reported a child life program. Space for activities was provided by half of the general hospitals. Almost half of the respondents indicated they saw no need for a similar program, while one third indicated interest in developing a program.

At that time, the divergence of program names reflected a lack of coherent identity across programs but a shared interest in meeting the needs of the hospitalized child. The programs identified in children's hospitals came under a variety of different titles (see accompanying table).[38] However, it would not be long before these diverging programs began to converge.

Dombro bemoaned the reality demonstrated by his data: "There are still too many hospitals that do not believe that the hospitalization of a child merits the effort necessary to provide total care. There are still too many hospitals that shun the family. Such conditions should not be tolerated, and they will not be if pediatricians and pediatric surgeons speak out and voice their displeasure."[40] Indeed, J. Alex Haller, M.D. of Johns Hopkins did speak out as editor of a collection of essays in *The Hospitalized Child and His Family* (1967). This publication was a milestone in the initiation of a "discussion of a child's relationship to and interaction with his hospital environment."[41] The compilation of professional perspectives on the effects of hospitalization on children, preparation for surgery, living-in arrangements for a parent, the importance of play for hospitalized children, and posthospitalization reactions and care, presented in union with Dombro's data on existing child life programs, offered a well-defined message: *total care* for pediatric patients and their families included provisions for play and preparation as a component of standard practice.

During this period, advances were made across all aspects of pediatric healthcare in North America. The formation of the Association for the Care of Children in Hospital and the complementary advances in play and education programs during the 1970s reflected a growing interest and respect for children. The concept of play as a right for children was on its way to becoming a core tenet of pediatric care.

Children's Activity Department
Children's Activity Service
Child Care
Child Development Unit—School, Extracurricular Activities
Formal Education—Preschool
Group Activities Department
Group Work Program—Intramural School
Institutional School—House Parent Recreation
Play Program—School, Recreational Activities
Recreational Department—Play Lady Program
Recreation Program—Play School
Rehabilitation—Recreation Program, Residential Treatment Department
Special Education Program
Special Education—Recreation Program

Additional titles in the survey for general hospitals included: [39]
Children's Ward Association
Educational-Recreational Therapy
Friends of the Hospital
Pediatric Education Program
Play Program—Day Care Centre
Recreation Therapy, School-Occupational Therapy
Special Education Program
Volunteer Services
Ward School
Play Program

ENDNOTES

1 Jack Rutkowski, A Survey of Child Life Programs, in *Child Life Activities: An Overview*, ed. Association for the Care of Children's Health, (Washington, DC: ACCH, 1978), 12.

2 Ibid.

3 Steven M. Spencer, We're Taking Better Care of Children Now, *The Saturday Evening Post*, (July 12, 1947); Jerome Ellison, They Heal Heartsick Children, *The Saturday Evening Post*, (July 30, 1955).

4 *Saturday Evening Post* (1947): 32.

5 Ibid.

6 Random House, *Little Golden Books Timeline*, Random House Kids, http://www.randomhousekids.com/brand/little-golden-books/timeline/

7 American Medical Association, Report on Historical Links Between the American Medical Association and the Hill-Burton Act, *American Medical Association Resources*, http://www.ama-assn.org/resources/doc/ethics/hillburton.pdf

8 n.a., Winnipeg's Children's Hospital, *The Canadian Hospital*, (October 1957): 37-58.

9 Winnipeg Children's Hospital, 43.

10 Winnipeg Children's Hospital, 38.

11 Bakwin, H., Loneliness in Infants, *American Journal of Diseases of Children*, *63* (1941): 30-40.

12 René A. Spitz, Hospitalism—An Inquiry into the Genesis of Psychiatric Conditions in Early Childhood, *Psychoanalytic Study of the Child*, *1*, (1945): 53-74.

13 Dane G. Prugh, Elizabeth M. Straub, Harriet H. Sands, Ruth M. Kirschbaum, and Ellenora A. Lenihan, A Study of the Emotional Reactions of Children and Families to Hospitalization and Illness, *American Journal of Orthopsychiatry*, *23*, (1953): 70-106.

14 Susan Pond Wojtasik and Claire White, The Story of Child Life, in *The Handbook of Child Life*, ed. Richard H. Thompson, (Springfield: Charles C. Thomas, 2009), 7.

15 Grace Langdon, "A Study of the Uses of Toys in a Hospital," *Child Development*, *19*(4), (1948): 197-212.

16 Claudia Gips, A Study of Toys for Hospitalized Children, *Child Development*, *21*(3), (1950): 149-161.

17 Grace Langdon, 207.

18 Ibid.

19 Grace Langdon, 208.

20 Ibid., 204. Note: Langdon noted the limitations of the exploratory study and suggested further study be undertaken.

21 Claudia Gips.

22 Claudia Gips, 156.

23 Ibid., 157.

24 Claudia Gips, 159.

25 Committee on Hospitals and Dispensaries of American Academy of Pediatrics, The Care of Children in Hospitals: Report of Committee on Hospitals and Dispensaries of American Academy of Pediatrics, *Pediatrics*, *14*, (1954): 413.

26 Burma Whitted and Roland B. Scott, The Significance of a Play Program in the Care of Children in a General Hospital, *Journal of the National Medical Association*, *54*(4), (1962): 488.

27 Ibid., 491.

28 Eleanor Blumgart and Barbara Maria Korsch, Pediatric Recreation: An Approach to Meeting the Emotional Needs of Hospitalized Children, *Pediatrics*, *34*, (1964): 133-136.

29 Veronica B. Tisza and Kristine Angoff, A Play Program and Its Function in a Pediatric Hospital, (Utica, NY: Utica College, Child Life Council Archives, January 1956).

30 Tisza and Angoff, 2.

31 Tisza and Angoff, 6.

32 Ibid.

33 Robert H. Dombro, Appendix A: Child Life Programs in Ninety-One Children's Hospitals in the United States and Canada, in *The Hospitalized Child and His Family*, ed. by J. Alex Haller, James L. Talbert, and Robert H. Dombro, (Baltimore: The Johns Hopkins Press, 1967).

34 Robert H. Dombro, Appendix B: Child Life Programs in Ninety-Two Pediatric Departments of General Hospitals in the United States and Canada, in *The Hospitalized Child and His Family*, ed. by J. Alex Haller, James L. Talbert, and Robert H. Dombro, (Baltimore: The Johns Hopkins Press, 1967).

35 Dombro, Appendix A, 90.

36 Ibid., 93

37 Dombro, Appendix B.

38 Dombro, Appendix A, 93.

39 Dombro, Appendix B, 107.

40 Ibid., 86.

41 J. Alex Haller, The Helen Schnetzer Child Life Program, in *The Hospitalized Child and His Family*, ed. by J. Alex Haller, James L. Talbert, and Robert H. Dombro, (Baltimore: The Johns Hopkins Press, 1967), v.

BIBLIOGRAPHY

Bakwin, H. Loneliness in Infants. *American Journal of Diseases of Children, 63*, (1941): 30-40.

Blumgart, Eleanor, & Korsch, Barbara Maria. Pediatric Recreation: An Approach to Meeting the Emotional Needs of Hospitalized Children. *Pediatrics, 34*, (1964): 133-136.

Committee on Hospitals and Dispensaries of American Academy of Pediatrics. The Care of Children in Hospitals: Report of Committee on Hospitals and Dispensaries of American Academy of Pediatrics. *Pediatrics, 14*, (1954): 413.

Dombro, Robert H. Appendix A: Child Life Programs in Ninety-One Children's Hospitals in the United States and Canada, in *The Hospitalized Child and His Family*, ed. by J. Alex Haller, James L. Talbert, and Robert H. Dombro (pp. 89-103). Baltimore: The Johns Hopkins Press, 1967.

Dombro, Robert H. Appendix B: Child Life Programs in Ninety-Two Pediatric Departments of General Hospitals in the United States and Canada, in *The Hospitalized Child and His Family*, ed. by J. Alex Haller, James L. Talbert, and Robert H. Dombro (pp. 105-117). Baltimore: The Johns Hopkins Press, 1967.

Ellison, Jerome. They Heal Heartsick Children. *The Saturday Evening Post*, (July 30, 1955).

Gips, Claudia. A Study of Toys for Hospitalized Children. *Child Development, 21*(3), (1950): 149-161.

Haller, J. Alex. The Helen Schnetzer Child Life Program, in *The Hospitalized Child and His Family*, edited by J. Alex Haller, James L. Talbert, and Robert H. Dombro (pp. 80-86). Baltimore: The Johns Hopkins Press, 1967.

Langdon, Grace. A Study of the Uses of Toys in a Hospital. *Child Development, 19*(4), (1948): 197-212.

n.a. Winnipeg's Children's Hospital. *The Canadian Hospital*, (October 1957).

Prugh, Dane G., Straub, Elizabeth M., Sands, Harriet H., Kirschbaum, Ruth M., & Lenihan, Ellenora A. A Study of the Emotional Reactions of Children and Families to Hospitalization and Illness, *American Journal of Orthopsychiatry*, *23*, (1953), 70-106.

Rutkowski, Jack. A Survey of Child Life Programs, in *Child Life Activities: An Overview*, edited by Association for the Care of Children's Health (pp. 11-15). Washington, DC: ACCH, 1978.

Spencer, Steven M. We're Taking Better Care of Children Now. *The Saturday Evening Post*, (July 12, 1947).

Spitz, René A. Hospitalism—An Inquiry into the Genesis of Psychiatric Conditions in Early Childhood. *Psychoanalytic Study of the Child*, *1*, (1945): 53-74.

Tisza, Veronica B., & Kristine Angoff. A Play Program and Its Function in a Pediatric Hospital. Utica, NY: Utica College, Child Life Council Archives, January 1956.

Whitted, Burma, & Scott, Roland B. The Significance of a Play Program in the Care of Children in a General Hospital. *Journal of the National Medical Association*, *54*(4), (1962): 488-491.

Wojtasik, Susan Pond, & White, Claire. The Story of Child Life, in *The Handbook of Child Life*, ed. by Richard H. Thompson (pp. 3-22). Springfield: Charles C. Thomas, 2009.

CHAPTER 4

A New Attitude in Using Play: Anne Smith

Joan Turner, *Mount Saint Vincent University*

"Please return to me unless you wish to keep it in the files as probably the earliest statement re Child Life. M.M.B. 1/85."

There is a solitary report located in Box 3, Folder 4 Hospitals/Play—1937 Report (Anne Smith) in the Child Life Council Archives at Utica College, New York.[1] It is a photocopy of a 25-page typewritten report with a handwritten note in the top righthand corner. "Please return to me unless you wish to keep it in the files as probably the earliest statement re Child Life. M.M.B. 1/85." Later, someone noted and circled the date, 1937.

Who is this Anne Smith and what is her place in the archives of child life? A close reading of the *Report on the Development of Play at the Children's Memorial Hospital, Chicago, Illinois* (CMHC) provides clues about Anne Smith—her understanding of group play, her values, and her commitment to the dissemination of knowledge of hospital play. The report provides a detailed cross section of the developing play program and related services as well as the circumstances of the Children's Hospital during the Great Depression, but little of the person Anne Smith. Further exploration of existing documents, however, reveals her to have been a practitioner actively engaged in research, scholarship, and advocacy during a time of shifting attitudes and practices within the child welfare movement. Indeed, a review of this early documentation of hospital-based play indicates that Anne Smith represents a previously unrecognized authority in the field of play for convalescing children.

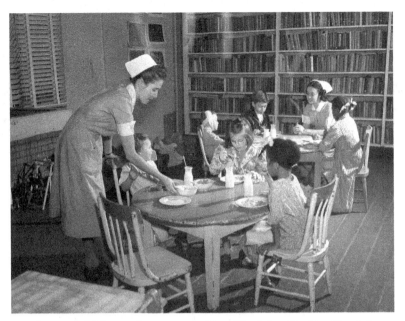

Group of children and nurses at mealtime, The Johns Hopkins Hospital
The Alan Mason Chesney Medical Archives of The Johns Hopkins Medical Institutions. Used with Permission.

A simple sketch, crafted following an examination of Smith's scholarly publications, the history of CMHC and related documents, situates the work of Anne Smith circa 1930s. Post-WW I and the Great Depression created challenging economic conditions for hospitals across the country. Outcomes following WWI served to direct attention to the unique needs of children as well as underscore the necessity of providing services for children early in life as a way to guarantee the next generation of healthy adults. Preventive medicine was a top priority resulting in the development of new initiatives across child welfare institutions, including children's hospitals.[2] The 1930 White House Conference on Child Health and Protection inspired what Anne Smith referred to as a "new attitude in using play" by drawing attention to the need for focused efforts supporting the care and condition of children.[3] Through a combination of a fiscally responsible administration and the acceptance of responsibilities that included the human side of a hospital, CMHC created an environment where play was embraced as a component of preventive medicine.[4]

Reliance on creative projects and fundraising was high during this period. "While at times in the Depression it seemed virtually impossible to run a top-quality hospital, that same period saw quality care, joined to love and concern for the 'whole' child, become the hallmark of Children's Memorial Hospital."[5] The context of fiscal gravity was exacerbated by an increase in free care. In 1935, the rate of what Smith referred to as "charity patients" was reported at 97%.[6] High unemployment, increased need for relief agencies, and rising costs over all were compounded as the market rate for endowments and the number of private bequests were reduced. The Auxiliary Board, responsible for managing the internal affairs of the hospital, and the Junior Auxiliary, mandated in a variety of areas related to volunteerism and special programs, were responsible for many of the social services provided for children and families. Hence, programs focused on the care of children (e.g., education, occupation, and recreation) were beginning to be recognized for their potential as complementary supports for nursing, medicine, and administrative agendas.

The introduction of the experimental play program noticeably addressed specific recommendations arising from the American Academy of Pediatrics Report on the Committee of Hospitals and Dispensaries: nurses training, preventive medicine, and the provision of care for convalescent children.[7,8] Led by an administration keeping an eye on the examination and reevaluation of programs and services, as well as maintaining Children's personality,[9] the need for a trained education and recreation worker was identified as a way to address some of the gaps. Given the fiscal realities at CMHC and Chief of Staff Dr. Joseph Brenneman's dedication to both an atmosphere of care and the validation of new interventions,[10] the evidence presented in the final report of the play experiment was likely valued by the hospital administration. As superintendent, Miss Binner would respond to considerations around the cost, space, and materials required for the play program relative to the impact on the quality of patient care.[11] Similarly, the principal of the training school and director of nursing, Miss Howe, would focus her attention on those efforts aimed at the extension of nurses training in areas such as play techniques, child development, child psychology and behavior, and the increased efficiency of nursing care. The Junior Auxiliary would also realize the benefit of enhanced recruitment and training of their volunteers for programs within a variety of settings in the hospital. In fact, the reputation of CMHC with the children is said to have been enhanced through the provision of the play program, "Our fame has grown, for the children spread the word, 'they play with you here.'"[12]

In 1932, the full-time play program was started. Limited volunteer-based entertainment had been provided during the 1920s but the Junior Auxiliary "soon realized that children needed more than story reading, coloring books and cutouts."[13] With the help of Neva Boyd, then assistant professor of sociology at

Northwestern University, Miss Anne Smith was selected and hired. The Junior Auxiliary paid a salary up to $100 per month, a respectful amount in light of the salary of the head resident at $100 per month, as reported by McCausland.[14] Described as Boyd's "student protégée" by Paru,[15] the selection of Smith is consistent with Binner's judgment, "Good service cannot be given unless the personnel are carefully selected. This is true in any hospital; it is doubly true in a children's institution."[16] Smith's association with Boyd suggests she came to CMHC with a background in group play and recreation. Indeed, Smith contributed to one of Boyd's publications, *Hospital and Bedside Games* (1919) as a result of her work with sick soldiers at Camp Custer, in Battle Creek, Michigan.[17,18] Later, Smith would dedicate her book, *Play for Convalescent Children in Hospital and at Home*, to Neva Boyd.[19] Although the specifics of Smith's educational background remain unknown, Boyd's recommendation is an indicator of qualifications commensurate with the demands of the position.[20]

According to Smith, group play throughout the day and evenings quickly became an accepted procedure. Determined to correct "faulty conceptions of play" she advanced theory and methods related to group play throughout the hospital.[21] Play was valued both as a form of preventive medicine and as a means of social adjustment: Smith stressed group play over individual play and active play over passive play. She advocated for cooperative play; rejected the presence of "artificial aides" such as prizes, rewards, and party favors; and rebuffed "commercial busy work." The play opportunities were provided from morning to evening in various locations. Play leaders included trained student nurses, field workers from Northwestern University, and volunteers. The increased visibility of children at play resulted in observations documented in nurses' notes such as the following example: "With a day filled with adequate play the hospitalized child is pleasantly fatigued and ready for a night's rest at an early hour. Better co-operation is secured from the child who is 'play satisfied' and the nurse's work is facilitated."[22]

By training nurses, staff, and volunteers, Smith was ensuring the longevity of this new approach to hospital play beyond her 6-year tenure. Smith openly criticized gratuitous play and a focus on play materials ("playthings do not constitute play") as she accelerated the professional training of play leaders.[23] Training in play techniques, particularly those that required no materials, were rooted within a hospital culture not only focused on fiscal restraint but also on the human side of care. Evidence of the shared responsibility of the whole staff for "making children happy and for preventing the development of fears" can be found across CMHC-related documents circa 1930s. For example, ward play was an expectation during evening nursing care: "nurses were encouraged to play with the children while giving routine physical care, to sing with them, to give them riddles or finger plays, guessing or sensing games, and to provide toys, books, or concentration materials before leaving the room."[24]

Certainly, Smith was the model for the new attitude of using play. The Children's play director was also engaged in direct patient care. Over a 6-day, 50-hour work-week her time with children was divided among preoperative play in the mornings followed by general duty on the wards where group play activity was facilitated. For Smith, the provision of play for hospitalized children was an exercise in exploration. Starting from a foundation in group play and an understanding of the procedures and living conditions for children in hospital, she proceeded to introduce activities in order to discover their potential for improving the conditions of children there. In her effort to avert negative outcomes, Smith emphasized recognition and exposition of those aspects of hospitalization and illness deemed most challenging for the children. Through the description of changes introduced to improve and generate more normal conditions for children she created a contrast with the traditional practices of the past as observed in the following excerpt: "At the end of three months, this practice of having orthopedic children wait near the operating room was discontinued. Thereafter these children waited in their own familiar wards and were played with until they were summoned, a plan more conducive to good morale."[25]

Careful documentation of summary data provided a record of the growing diversity of the activities of the play department for the years 1932 to 1937, including the introduction of play before minor operations, major operations, on the wards and in waiting areas, as well as educational displays, nature study, kindergarten, grade school instruction, the children's library, the nurses' library, and instruction in play.

The training of nurses, volunteers, staff, as well as colleagues visiting from children's hospitals spread the new attitude in using play throughout and beyond CMHC. The training of nurses and volunteers took place during the children's rest time, after which group play led by nurses and volunteers was also under her supervision. During 1932, Smith documented teaching six beginners' classes in play of 8 hours each, to a total of 205 affiliate nurses. In 1937, she documented teaching from six to eight classes per week as well as special classes to organize play equipment, an introductory and beginners' course to 84 staff nurses, and the supervision of affiliate nurses in a week of play on the wards. Descriptions and data presented in the report chronicle the extent of training presented in both the beginners' class in play and the advanced work in play class.[26] Over the course of the experiment 1,004 nurses received training in techniques of play—over 200 nurses came every year from all parts of the United States and Canada for practical training. The training component of the hospital play experiment alone suggests the pioneering role of Anne Smith in the development of hospital play programs.

Moreover, Smith's play program became both a model and a conduit for training for developing programs. Programs in children's institutions in Montreal, San Francisco, and South Euclid, for example, benefited from her contribution to the organization of recreational programs.[27] Many of the Northwestern University students who had completed their field training at CMHC went on to roles at other children's facilities including Cook County Hospital (Chicago), Boston Children's Hospital, and Children's Hospital in Denver, to name just a few.[28]

Although Paru suggested "[s]omething happened because work with groups all but disappeared from Children's when Anne Smith left in 1938,"[29] McCausland indicates, "[t]he Hospital's commitment to play therapy for its patients deepened as the years passed."[30] In fact, McCausland refers to Smith as "the Director of Recreation" in 1932—a title that stood long after her departure in 1937. Bernadine Kern is referred to as "the Recreation Director" in a publication dated 1939.[31] Much later, in 1976, the title was changed to "Child Life" under the direction of Myrtha Perez.[32] Indeed, even if rather anonymous, the legacy of Anne Smith cannot be denied.

Smith continued the dissemination of the knowledge gained from her experience at CMHC to a greater community over the next 25 years. In 1935–1936 she presented papers on group play in a hospital at two national conferences and at the Chicago Chapter of Social Workers Play Institute of the Child, and published two articles on play. In 1941, *Play for Convalescent Children in Hospital and at Home* made its début. Book reviews endorsing her work were published in leading medical journals.[33] Even after Smith had moved on from CMHC, her book remained popular as evidenced in a letter to Neva Boyd dated 1951, Evanston, Illinois. Here, Smith described her efforts to reprint the book in order to meet an international interest: "…requests keep coming. One via air mail came from Sydney, Australia; another from an army officer in Japan; one from Nat'l Infantile Association of Nw York [sic]."[34] Eventually the second edition was published in 1961. In addition to a new chapter on play in clinics where she used the title "play lady" Smith aligned her work with the developing field of recreation and the Council for the Advancement of Hospital Recreation.

Evidently, Smith moved on from play with convalescent children and continued her work in community recreation. By the time the first edition of her book was published, Smith was the staff instructor at Leaders' Training School, Community Recreation Service, in Chicago. Papers from the Neva Boyd Archive indicated activity in Evanston, Illinois, in the late 1940s where Smith prepared a report on the community use of the school as a recreation center. In this report, she advocated for neighborhood play centers where not only play space was a necessity but also play leaders trained with group play methods. Similar to the CMHC play experiment, this effort advocated for the training of play leaders and utilized a unique approach to university and community cooperation. A decade later, Smith was identified with three Minneapolis public health clinics and the Kenny Institute where again she lead an experiment with group play that was reported in the second edition of her book.[35]

Thus ends the trail of Miss Anne Smith. Based on the existing evidence, Smith had followed the path of recreation starting around 1918 working with wounded soldiers. Just as the child life profession began to take shape during the 1960s, her 40-plus-year career must have been coming to a close. Aside from the report on play described in *The Handbook of Child Life*,[36] the name Anne Smith has not made it into the common history of the child life profession. Although cited by Emma Plank,[37] additional indication of any connection to the emerging child life leaders has yet to be uncovered. To be sure, Anne Smith represents a previously unrecognized authority in the field of play for convalescing children. As a practitioner, researcher, and scholar, Anne Smith created a record of early play programs in hospitals that was shared internationally and contributed to the establishment of organized play for convalescing children.

ENDNOTES

1 Anne Smith, *Report on the Development of Play at Children's Memorial Hospital, Chicago Il,* (Utica, NY: Utica College, Child Life Council Archives, 1937).

2 Clare McCausland, *An Element of Love: A History of The Children's Memorial Hospital of Chicago, Il* (Chicago: The Children's Memorial Hospital, 1981), 96.

3 Anne Smith, *Play for Convalescent Children in Hospital and at Home,* (New York: A.S. Barnes and Company, 1941), 1.

4 Ibid., 4.

5 McCausland, *An Element of Love,* 98.

6 Smith, *Play for Convalescent Children in Hospital and at Home,* 45.

7 McCausland, *An Element of Love,* 96.

8 Clifford Grulee, Murray Bass, L.R. DeBuys, Roger Dennett, Henry Dietrich, Lewis Webb Hill, and George Munns, Report of the Committee on Hospitals and Dispensaries Social Service: Supplementary Report General Summary, *Journal of Pediatrics,* 6(2), (1935): 129-145.

9 Joseph Brennemann, The Children's Memorial Hospital, Chicago, *Journal of Pediatrics,* *4*(4), (1934): 528.

10 Stanley Gibson, Joseph Brennemann (1872–1944), *Journal of Pediatrics, 45*(6), (1954).

11 Mabel W. Binner, They Play with You Here, *The Modern Hospital, 44*(2), (1935): 54-58.

12 Smith, *Report on the Development of Play,* 3.

13 McCausland, *An Element of Love,* 58.

14 Ibid., 112.

15 Marden Paru, The Work of Anne Smith and Neva Boyd, Neva Leona Boyd Papers, (Chicago: University of Illinois Chicago Archives, 1965).

16 Binner, They Play with You Here, 55.

17 Paru, The Work of Anne Smith and Neva Boyd.

18 Neva L. Boyd, *Hospital and Bedside Games,* (Chicago: Neva L. Boyd, 1919).

19 Smith, *Play for Convalescent Children in Hospital and at Home.*

20 Note: Acknowledgment to Janine Zabriskie for her research at the University of Illinois Chicago Archives, Chicago. IL. Neva Leona Boyd Papers.

21 Smith, *Play for Convalescent Children in Hospital and at Home,* xiii.

22 Smith, *Report on the Development of Play,* 9.

23 Ibid., 6.

24 Ibid., 5.

25 Ibid., 3-24.

26 Ibid., 22.

27 Smith, *Report on the Development of Play at Children's Memorial Hospital, Chicago Il,* 22.

28 Smith, *Report on the Development of Play at Children's Memorial Hospital, Chicago Il,* 23.

29 Paru, *The Work of Anne Smith and Neva Boyd,* 13.

30 McCausland, *An Element of Love,* 104.

31 Bernadine Kern, How to Organize a Play Department in the Hospital, *Hospital Management,* (1939): np.

32 McCausland, *An Element of Love,* 178.

33 For example, *The Journal of Nervous and Mental Disease, American Journal of Public Health Nations Health* and *American Journal of Physical Medicine and Rehabilitation.*

34 Anne Smith, Letter to Leona Boyd, Neva Leona Boyd Papers, (Chicago: University of Illinois Chicago Archives, 1951).

35 Anne Smith, *Play for Convalescent Children in Hospital and at Home* (2nd edition), (New York: A.S. Barnes and Company, 1961).

36 Susan Pond Wojtasik and Claire White, The Story of Child Life, in *The Handbook of Child Life; A Guide for Pediatric Psychosocial Care,* ed. by Richard H. Thompson (pp. 3-22), (Illinois: Charles C. Thomas, 2009).

37 Emma Plank, *Working with Children in Hospitals,* (Cleveland: Western Reserve University, 1962), 105.

BIBLIOGRAPHY

Binner, Mabel W. They Play with You Here. *The Modern Hospital*, *44*(2), (1935): 54-58.

Boyd, Neva L. *Hospital and Bedside Games*. Chicago: Neva L. Boyd, 1919.

Brennemann, Joseph. The Children's Memorial Hospital, Chicago. *Journal of Pediatrics*, *4*(4), (1934): 528.

Gibson, Stanley. Joseph Brennemann (1872–1944). *Journal of Pediatrics*, *45*(6), (1954).

Grulee, Clifford G., Bass, Murray H., DeBuys, L. R., Dennett, Roger H., Dietrich, Henry, Webb Hill, Lewis, & Munns, George F. Report of the Committee on Hospitals and Dispensaries Social Service: Supplementary Report General Summary. *Journal of Pediatrics*, *6*(2), (1935): 129-145.

Kern, Bernadine. How to Organize a Play Department in the Hospital. *Hospital Management*, (April 1939): np.

McCausland, Clare. *An Element of Love: A History of The Children's Memorial Hospital of Chicago, Il*. Chicago: The Children's Memorial Hospital, 1981.

Paru, Marden. The Work of Anne Smith and Neva Boyd, Neva Leona Boyd Papers. Chicago: University of Illinois Chicago Archives, 1965.

Plank, Emma. *Working with Children in Hospitals*. Cleveland: Western Reserve University, 1962.

Smith, Anne. *Report on the Development of Play at Children's Memorial Hospital, Chicago Il*. Utica, NY: Utica College, Child Life Council Archives, 1937.

Smith, Anne. *Play for Convalescent Children in Hospital and at Home*. New York: A.S. Barnes and Company, 1941.

Smith, Anne. Letter to Leona Boyd, Neva Leona Boyd Papers. Chicago: University of Illinois Chicago Archives, 1951.

Smith, Anne. *Play for Convalescent Children in Hospital and at Home* (2nd ed). New York: A.S. Barnes and Company, 1961.

Wojtasik, Susan Pond, & White, Claire. The Story of Child Life. In *The Handbook of Child Life; A Guide for Pediatric Psychosocial Care*, ed. by Richard H. Thompson (pp. 3-22). Illinois: Charles C. Thomas, 2009.

CHAPTER 5

Play as a Right: B.J. Seabury (1927–2002)

Lois Pearson, *School of Education at Edgewood College*

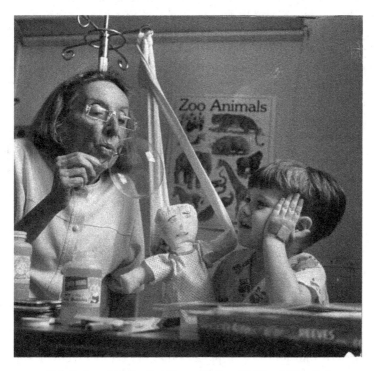

B. J. Seabury blowing bubbles at Hasbro Children's Hospital
Reprinted by Permission, Marianne Cooney, Rhode Island Hospital/ Hasbro Children's Hospital

Dr. Edwin Forman, a pediatrician on the staff at Rhode Island Children's Hospital, recalls the moment when he first met B.J. in 1976. "I introduced myself and said, 'I understand that you are our Play Therapist.' She gave me a sharp look and in a voice that I could tell even then was one to be reckoned with, answered, 'I'm not a therapist. Play isn't just for diagnosis or therapy. It's these children's right and their need.'"[1] Described as a diminutive child life pioneer, her statement of play as a right became the cornerstone of her career and the heart of her passion.

The photo opening this chapter could not be more appropriate for introducing Barbara-Jeanne Seabury. "She can often be found talking with a parent or trying her skill with a jar of bubbles to the delight of a Potter patient."[2] The principle of a child's right to play is the focus of the story of B.J. Seabury. Not unusual for women of her time, B.J. had a lifetime of careers. Starting in early childhood education, her progression from kindergarten teacher to a recognized leader working with children with disabilities positioned B.J. as an advocate for vulnerable children. In association with educational programs at Smith College and the University of Massachusetts in the early 1960s, she developed a reputation as a policymaker for change in childcare and education. Eventually her pioneering role in early hospital play programs in and around Boston, and back to Rhode Island, contributed to the emerging focus on the right of children to play as a standard of care for children in hospitals. Certainly her tiny stature belied the strength of her convictions about play for children in every setting.

B.J. as a Teacher and Learner

B.J.'s passion for children and their developmental needs advanced over time. Her bachelor of science degree from the University of Rhode Island (1940) was in child development and family relations, with a minor in psychology and education. After graduation, she quickly found her first job as a kindergarten teacher in the Providence Public Schools for 4 years. Young teachers like B.J. were easily captivated by the play of young children in the kindergarten classroom; for B.J., it seemed that the observation of young 5-year-olds developing a more complex understanding and ability to engage in cooperative play sensitized her to the importance of play. Although there is little information about her decision to move to Evansville, Indiana, one can speculate that an early interest in play and development propelled her into work with vulnerable children.

In the early 1950s, the outlook for children with disabilities was dismal. Children were either placed in institutions or remained at home but were not accepted into the public school system.[3] Therefore, anyone with an interest in working with children with disabilities found themselves employed away from the mainstream educational system, for example in rehabilitation centers. In 1952, B.J. became the program coordinator and head teacher at the Vanderburgh County Society for Crippled Children and Adults founded in 1946 (later known as the Rehabilitation Center of Evansville).[4] The preschool center for children was opened in 1950 in a Quonset hut on the campus of Evansville College. After B.J. began her work in 1952, she moved into the roles of program coordinator, head teacher, and eventually director of volunteer services (1952–1959).[5] During her 7 years of work there, the center built a new facility, the first in the United States designed solely for the purpose of outpatient rehabilitation. Given the state of education for children with disabilities and the lack of knowledge regarding the importance of socialization, one could conclude that B.J. had a hand in the creation of the new environment highlighting opportunities for play as a strong element of programming. Viewed as an expert on children with special needs, B.J. recalled that she worked in physical, occupational, and speech therapy and did social work. "This had a profound effect on me...working with these children."[6]

After almost 8 years at the Rehabilitation Center of Evansville, eventually the Easter Seal Society of Southwestern Indiana, B.J. had established a strong foundation of programming for handicapped children. During this period in Evansville, B.J. completed her master of arts degree in education at Eastern Michigan University (1956), but she was also becoming disheartened. While her skills as a leader had been recognized and embraced, she missed working directly with the children and began searching for other opportunities.[7]

B.J. as an Educator

B.J. returned to the East Coast in 1959, to find herself in the best of both worlds as an educator for emerging child development experts and also with young children in the preschool. As a faculty resident at Smith College in Massachusetts, B.J. taught courses on child development and working with children with special needs. Always the consummate educator, she also served as the lead teacher of the Laboratory Nursery School and taught a child development course at the University of Massachusetts at Amherst.[8]

Given B.J.'s lifelong passion for teaching, one does wonder why, at this stage of her career she became so interested in children in hospitals. Perhaps she began to recognize gaps in the care of the young handicapped children with whom she worked; perhaps her teaching at Smith College and the University of Massachusetts had exposed her to like-minded leaders in child development and pediatrics. Her position in an academic institution likely exposed her to new knowledge and experts to support a transition into new areas of interest. At that time, children with disabilities were most often medically fragile and faced frequent hospitalizations, medical procedures, and treatments. For example, children born with spina bifida had only a 10% to 12% survival rate[9] while polio had reached epidemic proportions in the United States and survivors constituted one of the largest groups of children with disabilities.[10] The classic study by Prugh, Staub, Sands, Kirschbaum, and Lenihan (1953), described not only the psychological distress of hospitalized children but also elucidated potential interventions to ameliorate the hospital environment to better support children and their families.[11]

As recalled by Marianne Cooney in her Memorial Service Remarks, B.J. was deeply troubled to discover "traumatic conditions" for children in hospitals.[12] Most disturbing to the recovery of children, B.J. thought, was the treatment of parents in the hospital setting. Parents were routinely subjected to limited "allowed" visiting hours which were strictly followed with the firm conviction that children were better off without the upset that frequently occurred when parents were present. The transition to healthcare seemed to be a natural one for B.J. Given her educational preparation and experience up to this point, B.J. was able to introduce change to improve the care and conditions for children and families in the hospital setting.

When a position opened at the Children's Hospital Medical Center of Boston, B.J. accepted the challenge to start an activities program involving play, school, and support for parents of hospitalized children. Her title was recreation coordinator, and she spent 3 years in the position. Evelyn Hausslein (Wheelock College, retired) came to work with B.J. in 1961 and immediately noted the changes taking place. Evelyn commented that prior to B.J.'s arrival, there were play and activity *schedules*. The first thing that B.J. did was eliminate the schedule and replace it with free play available throughout the day. For B.J., play was not a four-letter word; she believed that every child deserved time to play, especially children who lived in the hospital.[13] B.J. stayed at the Children's Hospital Medical Center until 1964 at which point her career took another turn, this time toward mental health services.

Returning to the nursery school arena, but with a clinical twist, B.J. worked for the Massachusetts Department of Mental Health from 1964 to1966. She gained considerable influence at this level of authority and experience that positioned her for the next transition: this time to Washington, D.C.

B.J. as a Policy Maker

Play as a child's right continued to be the focus of B.J.'s work in her next career transition. She moved to Washington, D.C., in 1966, to become director of the National Child Research Center (NCRC), a position which she held for 5 years.[14] The NCRC had been founded in the late 1920s as a research facility; its mission included the engagement of outstanding faculty, opportunities for professional development, implementation of cutting-edge research, inclusion of children with special needs, a curriculum based on early childhood development, and parent education. During that time, the NCRC partnered with the National Institute of Health to conduct a major study of young children's social behavior and pioneered training for Head Start teachers in the Washington, D.C., area.

Stephanie Henry, B.J.'s niece and child life specialist in Connecticut, recalls that as the director of NCRC, B.J. was invited to a bill signing at the White House—an experience B.J. had described as "thrilling."[15] Although the exact bill was not clearly identified nor was the precise date, it was evidently part of President Lyndon Johnson's "Great Society," a series of domestic programs that included the War on Poverty and generated dozens of educational efforts for impoverished children and adults.[16] B.J. was part of the panel of child development experts who designed the creation of Project Head Start, a notable accomplishment of Johnson's presidency. Today, Head Start continues to provide poor and at-risk preschool children with a greater chance for success as they enter the public school system. A single photograph, circa 1967, has preserved evidence of B.J.'s contribution to Head Start.[17]

The photo held in the Child Life Council Historical Archives highlights B.J.'s sense of humor and continuous delight in all things childlike, by showing her presenting an oversized stuffed llama at the White House. The two-headed llama was actually a character named Pushmi-Pullyu, from the 1967 musical film based on the earlier series of Dr. Doolittle novels written by Hugh Lofting.[18] B.J. is standing next to Luci Baines Johnson, the president's youngest daughter, her tiny stature readily apparent. Conceivably, the photo represents B.J.'s assertion of the right to play—even at a White House function.

Finally, in 1971, B.J. returned to Boston and began the serious work of promoting child's play as director of children's activities services at Children's Hospital Medical Center. In this position she honed her skills of advocacy and brought attention to the importance of programming for families in the hospital setting. In a speech given at the 11th Annual Association for the Care of Children's Health (ACCH) Conference in Denver in 1976, entitled "Who Works for Children: The Realities," she shared, "I want to tell you some of the things we've been through at Children's in Boston, not because we've solved them perfectly, but because they've helped us learn."[19] She told tales of the renovation to the main playroom and the front lobby; changes to the work schedule; incorporation of activities specialists in admissions, clinics, and the emergency room; and the initiation of a dialogue on roles, professional self-perception, and perceptions of others. With each tale, B.J. shared a lesson, too. The first related to the timing of proposals—when to make them and when to combine strategies focused on the children and their needs. Secondly, she illustrated how professional groups did not need to be competitive, particularly when the mutual focus of their efforts was on the children and their needs.[20] Examples included the introduction of 24-hour visitation for parents, collaboration on the redesign of the hospital to make it more welcoming, activities for children in waiting areas, and options for using play to help understand hospital procedures—all designed to keep children engaged in play and to decrease anxiety.[21]

That same year, B.J. received a call from Dr. Leo Stern, then chief of pediatrics at Rhode Island Hospital and Brown University.[22] He wanted B.J. to return to her home state to start the first child life program in Rhode Island. B.J. had previously noted that many children and families chose to come to Boston for medical treatment, rather than to Rhode Island Hospital (RIH). She was lured by the promise and the challenge that RIH was ready to make changes necessary to provide the best pediatric care possible for the families of Rhode Island (1976–1993).

She arrived at RIH with a strong commitment to make those changes happen, saying, "[P]lay is not to be considered an oasis from treatment; it is actually a part of it."[23] Only a few months after her arrival, she told the board of directors, "If I had children who needed hospitalization, I would not bring them here."[24] Her intent was to effect change and she was ready to do so: "Children have so many needs when they are hospitalized aside from medicine."[25] The foundation of her beliefs were that (1) play served as a bridge between hospital and home, (2) play offered a chance to release tension, and (3) play provided a way to communicate, both verbally and nonverbally.[26] For B.J., even the choice *not* to play would allow children to take some control of their situation when so much else about the hospital experience offered no choices. Her first step was to open the previously unused hospital playrooms. She was intent on recognizing that siblings and parents also needed to be included in these experiences.

Special events programming, cooking, ice cream socials, and other activities were made available for children of all ages. These activities were introduced specifically to emphasize the importance of the social needs of the child: "A child's mental attitude is an inseparable part of the recovery process. If his attitude is good and he is intact emotionally, he is remarkably more responsive as a patient."[27] B.J. also recognized the distinct needs of adolescents. To that end, she started a teen center where youth could engage in conversation and developmentally appropriate activities with peers. A school program was also initiated by B.J. and despite much resistance and many struggles, continued to be an important part of pediatric programming. One young adolescent remarked, "I was convinced that I was going to die in the hospital until a hospital school teacher came to teach me about nouns and adverbs, and I thought, no one would bother to do that if I was really dying."[28]

B.J. in Summary

This chapter illustrated the accomplishments of B.J. Seabury up to the mid-1970s, particularly her commitment to honor the child's right to play in hospital. While these accomplishments were notable for the time, her impact also continued to be felt well into the 1990s. Many disciplines and awards have since recognized her advocacy for children in healthcare settings. As a leader in the formation of the Association for the Care of Children's Health (1967), she served as the president (1977–1979) in addition to taking on other roles such as chairwoman of the 10th Annual Conference and the special consultant for the 20th Annual Conference. She followed Emma Plank as the liaison to the American Academy of Pediatrics, Hospital Care Committee and served on the Editorial Advisory Committee for the journal *Children's Health Care* (1983–1989). Much later, she was a charter member of the Child Life Council, received the 1990 Distinguished Service Award, and was conferred an honorary degree of Doctor of Education from Wheelock College in 1994.

In the 1993 Emma Plank Keynote Address, "Child Life: Attitudes and Images," B.J. choose to remind members of the emerging profession, "If we want to move ahead, we must know what happened in the past—we must have a historical perspective. It is not true that nothing happened in child life until you went to work a couple of years ago."[29] The legacy of Barbara-Jean Seabury goes beyond her commitment to a child's right to play. Her enduring message was also about collaboration and the importance of maintaining a focus on the needs of the child across disciplines. Evelyn Hausslein summed up B.J.'s accomplishments best when she commented on her work with B.J. at Children's Hospital of Boston: "When I saw play as an activity, B.J. saw it as essential to a child's development."[30]

ENDNOTES

1 Edwin N. Forman, Letter of Recognition for B. J. Seabury, *Special Awards for Lifetime Achievements in Child Life*, (Utica, NY: Child Life Council Archives, May 1990).
2 n.a., The Power of One Child Life's: B. J. Seabury Receives National Recognition, (Utica, NY: Child Life Council Archives).
3 The History of Special Education in the United States, Special Education News, http://www.specialednews.com/the-history-of-special-education-in-the-united-states.htm
4 Easter Seals Rehabilitation Center – A History, http://in-sw.easterseals.com/site/PageServer?pagename=INSW_whoweare
5 Barbara-Jeanne Seabury, Curriculum Vitae, (Utica, NY: Child Life Council Archives, June 1994).
6 Litchfield, Kathy, SK Woman Honored for Helping Children, *The Narragansett Times*, *29*, (April 1994): 4-A.
7 Ibid.
8 Seabury, Curriculum Vitae.
9 Lisa Pruitt, Living with Spina Bifida: A Historical Perspective, *Pediatrics*, *130*(2), (February 2012): 181-183. http://pediatrics.aappublications.org/content/130/2/181.extract
10 http://www.historyofvaccines.org/content/timelines/all
11 Dane G. Prugh, Elizabeth M. Staub, Harriet H. Sands, Ruth M. Kirschbaum, and Elenora A. Lenihan," A Study of the Emotional Reactions of Children and Families to Hospitalization and Illness, *The American Journal of Orthopsychatry*, *23*(1), (1953): 70-106.
12 Marianne Cooney, *Memorial Service Remarks*, (Providence, RI, 2002).
13 Evelyn Hausslein, Telephone conversation, April 4, 2013.
14 National Child Research Center, NCRC History, accessed February 7, 2013, http://ncrcpreschool.org/page.php?pid=93 ().
15 Stephanie J. Henry, Series of email communications with Lois Pearson, October 2013 to December 2013.
16 http://www.acf.hhs.gov/programs/ohs/about/history-of-head-start
17 Child Life Council Historical Archives, (Utica, NY). Note: unfortunately, the photograph is not documented for copyright access and therefore is not available for print in this publication.

18 Doctor Doolittle, http://etc.usf.edu/lit2go/221/the-story-of-doctor-dolittle.

19 Barbara-Jeanne Seabury, Who Works for Children: The Realities, *Journal of The Care of the Association for the Care of Children in Hospitals*, 5(3), (1977): 12.

20 Seabury, Who Works for Children: The Realities, 17.

21 S. Clatworthy, Therapeutic Play: Effects on Hospitalized Children, *Journal of Association for the Care of Children's Health*, 9(4), (1981): 108-113.

22 Rhode Island Hospital, Our New Activities Program: Meeting the Needs of Children and Adolescents, *Nite Lite*, (Providence: Rhode Island Hospital, September 1976), np.

23 Ibid.

24 Wayne Worchester, B-J Cares Enough to Help Kids in Hospital, *Providence Journal*, (1977).

25 Kathy Litchfield, SK Woman Honored for Helping Children, *The Narragansett Times*, 29, (April 1994): 4-A.

26 Rhode Island Hospital, Our New Activities Program.

27 Wayne Worchester, B-J Cares Enough to Help Kids in Hospital.

28 Beverley H. Johnson, Elizabeth Seale Jeppson, and Lisa Redburn, *Caring for Children and Families: Guidelines for Hospitals*, (Bethesda, MD: Association for the Care of Children's Health, 1992), 394.

29 Barbara-Jeanne Seabury, The Child Life Profession: Attitudes and Images, *Emma Plank Keynote Address*, (Utica, NY: Child Life Council Archives), 8.

30 Evelyn Hausslein, Telephone conversation, April 14, 2013.

BIBLIOGRAPHY

Battle, Constance. Gene Stanford "Power of One" Award Presentation. Utica, NY: Child Life Council Archives.

Bolig, Rosemary. Guest Editorial: The Diversity of Play in Health Care Settings. *Children's Health Care*, 16(3), (1988): 132-133.

Bolig, Rosemary. Play in Health Care Settings: A Challenge for the 1990's. *Children's Health Care*, 19(4), (1990): 229-233.

Brazelton, T. Berry, & Thompson, R. Child Life. *Pediatrics*, 81(5), (1988): 725-726

Children's Hospital Boston. http://www.childrenshospital.org/bcrp/Site2213/mainpag-eS2213P1.html

Clatworthy, S. Therapeutic Play: Effects on Hospitalized Children. *Journal of Association for the Care of Children's Health*, 9(4), (1981): 108-113.

Cooney, Marrianne. *Memorial Service Remarks*. Providence, RI. Utica, NY: Child Life Council Archives, 2002.

Employee Update. Come Help Us Say Goodbye, BJ. Rhode Island Hospital. *Public Relations*, 5(6), (1993). Utica, NY: Child Life Council Archives.

Forman, Edwin N. Letter of Recognition for B. J. Seabury. *Special Awards for Lifetime Achievements in Child Life*. Utica, NY: Child Life Council Archives, May 1990.

Freyer, Felice. Woman Who Changed Hospital Life for Children Honored. *Providence Journal Bulletin*, 8, (February 1993).

Hassenfeld, Alan G. Celebrating the Life of B.J. Seabury. *The Providence Journal*, (May 17, 2002). www.projo.com

Henry, Stephanie J. Personal recollections of her aunt B.J., email. Personal papers of Lois Pearson.

Johnson, Beverley H., Seale Jeppson, Elizabeth, & Redburn, Lisa. *Caring for Children and Families: Guidelines for Hospitals*. Bethesda, MD: Association for the Care of Children's Health, 1992.

Litchfield, Kathy. SK Woman Honored for Helping Children. *The Narragansett Times*, (April 29, 1994): 4-A.

Pass, Marilynn, & Bolig, Rosemary. A Comparison of Play Behaviors in Two Child Life Program Variations. *Children's Health Care*, 22(1), (1993): 5-17.

Pruitt, Lisa. Living with Spina Bifida: A Historical Perspective. *Pediatrics, 130*(2) (2012): 181-183.

Rhode Island Hospital. Our New Activities Program: Meeting the Needs of Children and Adolescents. *Nite Lite*. Providence: Rhode Island Hospital, September 1976, np.

Seabury, Barbara-Jeanne. Curriculum Vitae. Utica, NY: Child Life Council Archives.

Seabury, Barbara-Jeanne. Who Works for Children: The Realities. *Journal of The Care of the Association for the Care of Children in Hospitals*, 5(3), (1977): 12-17.

Seabury, Barbara-Jeanne. The Child Life Profession: Attitudes and Images. *Emma Plank Keynote Address*. Utica, NY: Child Life Council Archives, 1993.

Severo, Richard. Play Eases the Fears of Hospitalized Children. *The New York Times*. http://www.newyorktimes/1981/06/09/science/play-eases-the-fears-of-hospitalized-children.html

Stillman, Diane. Help for Hospitalized Children. *McCalls Magazine*, (March 1990): 48.

Thompson, Richard H., & Stanford, Gene. *Child Life in Hospitals: Theory and Practice*. Springfield, IL: Charles Thomas, 1981.

Wilson, Jerrianne. Future of Play in Health Care Settings. *Children's Health Care, 16*(3), (1988): 231-237.

Worcester, Wayne. B-J Cares Enough to Help Kids in Hospital. *Providence Journal*, (1977).

CHAPTER 6

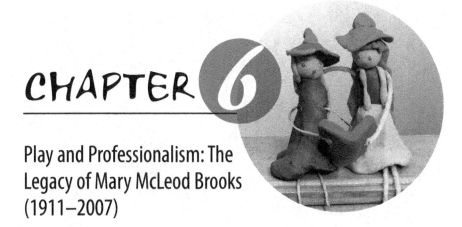

Play and Professionalism: The Legacy of Mary McLeod Brooks (1911–2007)

Civita Brown, *Utica College*

> *Play is a child's life, his work, his way of living.*[1]
> *"Humanizing healthcare for children..."*[2]
> *"Treating the total child..."*[3]

In the summer of 1977, I sat in a classroom listening to Dr. Gene Stanford lecturing, when I first heard the name of Mary Brooks. He told my class of two students (the first in our program) that Mary and Emma Plank were "the pioneers, the shapers, the molders, the builders" of the field of child life. Mary Brooks, he said, professed the importance of play for children who were hospitalized and stressed that those going into the field of child life must be educated and knowledgeable regarding development of healthy children, as well as children in the hospital. I continue to use the information from that lecture to teach my students about the significance of these two exceptional women to the field of child life. Mary Brooks referred to Emma Plank as "the godmother of child life," but she too oversaw, nurtured, advocated, and shaped the child life profession.

The phrases at the beginning of this chapter are synonymous with Mary Brooks's life and work. Mary's role in advocating for play and professionalism in the child life field can be traced from her early dreams of working with sick children through her days in Boston. In Boston, Mary discovered play in the hospital, started one of the first hospital play programs, and advocated for play in the pediatric milieu.

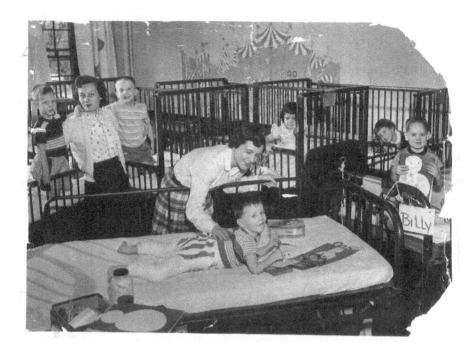

Six children take a break from activity with Junior League volunteers
Photo courtesy of the Junior League of Nashville, Tennessee.
Reprinted by Permission from the Junior League of Nashville Tennessee

Later she became an advocate for the education of hospital play and recreation workers, and finally she played a key role as one of the founding members of the Association for Care of Children in Hospitals.

Mary's love of children and play began early. Raised in a medicine-oriented family, her brothers both became doctors, and she dreamed of one day working with children in hospitals. As a child, she and her older brother frequently played "hospital." He operated on her dolls and she assisted as the nurse. According to Mary, her dolls were her life and she always envisioned a life devoted to working with children, particularly hospitalized children.

In 1933, Mary Brooks graduated from Smith College. The foreword to her senior yearbook says, "…to the class who saw the bad side of good times and the good side of bad times." A letter from the Child Life Council Archives dated May 6, 1988, reports that Mary felt she had been "programmed" for this prestigious college.[4] She was disappointed to realize that Smith would not be preparing "nurse girls," or even "nursery nurses," as universities did in Great Britain. In 1932, when she was a junior at Smith, she discovered a nursery school on campus.[5] That year, the play program at Children's Memorial Hospital of Chicago began under Anne Smith. An article by Mabel Binner described the program and discussed the effects of play preceding operations for children under treatment at the hospital, which laid the groundwork for the importance of play in the hospital.[6] After discovering the campus nursery school, Mary soon learned that nursery school teaching was a new but very respectable career. As she explained in the same letter, she quickly enrolled in a summer course at Vassar College, where she was introduced to pioneering teachers in the field that would become early childhood education. Her letter also describes two sisters, both graduates of the Boston Children's School of Nursing, who had gone on to study child development and early childhood education and who also strongly influenced her desire to teach nursery school. After graduation, Mary attended graduate school at the Merrill-Palmer Institute in Detroit, one of the best programs for early childhood education at the time, and later received a master's degree from Teacher's College of Columbia University. Mary went on to teach early childhood education at Berea College in Kentucky and Wheaton College in Illinois.

Mary eventually moved to Boston to teach in a nursery school, where she rekindled her friendship with Elizabeth (Sally) Staub. Mary and Sally met years earlier at a conference in Boston. They spent evenings together envisioning their ideal employment: working with a group of pediatricians or in a children's hospital. Mary attributed her strong and continuing interest in medicine to her brothers, who were then in medical school. In Mary's retelling, Sally's dream had finally been realized, and Sally had become involved in a research project at Children's Medical Center (now Children's Hospital Boston) with child psychiatrist Dane Prugh. In Mary's interview, she discussed how the Prugh research began to build the foundation for the new profession of child life. In 1953, Dr. Prugh, along with Sally Staub, Harriet Sands, Ruth Kirschbaum, and Ellenora Lenihan, initiated the first controlled study of the emotional effects of hospitalization on children and families at Children's Medical Center in Boston.[7] The experimental group of children received psychological preparation and support during procedures, liberal visiting hours for their families, earlier ambulation, a special play program, and greater involvement of their parents in their care on the ward. The control group received standard care, which included none of these interventions. Play was referred to as "education and recreation." Ultimately, the researchers determined that the experimental group demonstrated better adjustment to the hospital than the control group. Their study would subsequently be cited in many articles and books on play.

Upon completion of the study, Sally Staub returned to teaching nursery school in Rochester, New York. Soon after, in 1955, Mary was invited by Dr. Prugh to become the director of a program of therapeutic play at the Children's Hospital of Philadelphia (CHOP). Mary thought that the program's title of "Leisure Time Activities" was unfortunate and inappropriate, so she soon changed it to "Children's Activities." That same year, Emma Plank was asked by pediatrician Fred Robbins to create a program addressing the social, emotional, and educational needs of the hospitalized children at Cleveland City Hospital.

Luci Weber, CCLS, the former director of child life at All-Children's Hospital in St. Petersburg, Florida, met Mary upon her retirement to Clearwater, Florida. In their conversations, Mary reminisced about the early days of the program at Children's Hospital of Philadelphia. The storage space for toys, materials, and supplies was located several buildings away from CHOP, so Mary regularly took a cart, filled it with toys, and pushed it down the streets of Philadelphia to the hospital.[8] In a taped CLC History Committee interview, Mary recalled the history of the Children's Hospital of Philadelphia as the first children's hospital in the United States, founded in 1855 when physicians were just beginning to recognize that children had unique needs, distinct from adults. The hospital delegated the Board of Lady Visitors to "entertain and educate little patients."[9] She felt the board had built the foundation for her to begin a play program at CHOP a hundred years later. Mary also vividly described how old the hospital building already was when she began working there. Patients were still housed in open wards—in some ways, an advantage to her new program because the playroom was in the middle of the ward and visible to all the children, regardless of their condition. Interns, residents, physicians, and nurses could readily observe the children during their sessions, developing a better understanding of the importance of play. Mary recalled one nurse who told her that even one of the children who was supposedly "asleep," having just returned from surgery at the time of the activities, nonetheless told the nurse about the play lady the next day.

Mary was very proud of being called a "play lady." Journalist Nancy Burden wrote, in an article about Mary, "Pladylady, playlady, shouted the little boy in pajamas."[10] Mary stated cheerfully, "We go on as happy people." She explained, "Sometimes we decide, sometimes they decide and sometimes we decide together what we'll play that day. It might be a morning of painting, crayoning, playing blocks or fashioning figures with play dough. In general, we emphasize unstructured play because we feel it is best from the point of view of child development. It helps them work out their anxieties and project their concerns and misunderstandings. As these show up we can pick them up. Playing doctor particularly helps a child work out their fears."[11] Her staff at that time were referred to as play specialists, and were each paid approximately $6,500 as an annual starting salary, with a 5% increase each year. A director received approximately $10,000 annually.[12]

An article published in the *Philadelphia Enquirer* magazine on September 11, 1966, reported about "Toy Time."[13] It explained how hospital psychiatrists discovered valuable insights by watching children at play. Mary was featured in a picture with a young child blowing bubbles; both appeared to be truly enjoying the moment. At the time, the child life program at CHOP existed under the auspices of the psychiatry department, members of which also recognized the importance of play to children's mental health and development. In *Play for Hospitalized Children*, published in 1969, Mary described play as a tool for diagnosing a child's fears, anxieties, and concerns. She stressed the importance of play as a means of communicating with the child, as well as the way children naturally learn about their world. Play, she said, is children's daily work, the way a child "works out solutions to many things that puzzle him."[14] In writings on play from 1966 to 1976, Mary explained how play was crucial to intellectual growth, physical ability, social experience, and emotional development. She emphasized that children need to play because normal growth and development didn't cease when a child was hospitalized. She wrote, "…because play reduces anxiety, children will continue to play in a hospital just as they continue to play in bomb shelters and concentration camps."[15] *Play in the Hospital*, a film Mary authored in 1971, depicted a hospital pediatric play program and argued that professionally supervised play can alleviate the fears and anxieties of hospitalized children. The film showed children playing out their experiences during hospitalization and demonstrated how a well-designed play program could meet the psychosocial needs of hospitalized children while also assisting the pediatric staff in their understanding of the individual child—the whole child.[16] In *Why Play in the Hospital* (1970), Mary wrote about the importance of treating the whole child. She emphasized that a child does not come to the hospital with just an illness or injury, but brings along his family support, family situation, and previous experiences.[17]

Mary frequently wrote about misperceptions of the term "play" that to some evoked frivolous connotation. The child life profession continues to struggle with that misconception today. Physicians and nurses still tell child life specialists, "You *play* with children all day—wish I had such a cushy job." Mary was proud of the title "Play Lady" but she also understood that the child life field needed to develop a sense of professionalism in order to assist other health professionals in understanding the importance of play. Mary often discussed the concept of "humanizing" healthcare for children. She was truly one of the early and visionary voices of child life. She advocated for play for children and the education of child life workers, and her motto was, "Treating the total child."[18] She believed that having a love for children was not enough; child life specialists also had to have a respect for play as the work of children, as well as formal training in child development.[19] Between 1969 and 1976, Mary published many articles on play which were later cited in other articles as well as in *A Pediatric Play Program: Developing a Therapeutic Play Program for Children in Medical Settings* by Pat Azarnoff and Sharon Flegal (1975).[20]

Along with her passion for play, Mary focused on the need for child life programs to be supervised by professionally trained individuals with experience working with children. She was convinced that individuals needed to not only be able to work well with young children but also needed specialized training working specifically with children who were hospitalized. She also believed that anyone interested in working in the hospital setting needed the ability to work well under stress.[21,22]

Mary was frustrated that many early play programs were left under the supervision of untrained volunteers. Although she appreciated the contribution of volunteers to sometimes underfunded play programs, she also argued that a "highly skilled, professionally trained director is essential if play is to achieve its maximum potential in the overall program of child care."[23] Between the 1950s and early 1970s, it was difficult to find educated staff to work in child life programs, so Mary felt she had to push for more rigorous academic and clinical training. In the 1970s, colleges and universities finally began offering coursework in child life.

Mary also recognized the critical importance of interdisciplinary collaboration. She saw that working in collaboration with physicians, nurses, administrative personnel, occupational therapy, physical therapy, and social work would help to professionalize the field of child life. The formation of ACCH in 1965 created an organization open to all these disciplines and vocations, united in pursuit of better care of hospitalized children. Mary wrote about the importance of this interdisciplinary group to make "hospitalization a healthy experience for children."[24] She believed that the ACCH influenced play programs to become "more professional in nature with greater emphasis on the basic needs of children, less on mere entertainment and diversion."[25] She realized that the field also needed a truly professional title for individuals trained to work with children and families in the hospital. In the summer 1975 issue of the *Journal of the Association for the Care of Children in Hospitals*, Mary wrote, "The outdated title of 'Play Lady' will hopefully disappear as soon as we are able to find the elusive 'right' title for what is now being called Child Life/Recreation." [26]

Back in those early months in Philadelphia, Mary first met Emma Plank, who she fondly called "our dear Nuschi," at an orthopsychiatric meeting. Mary immediately recognized the similarities between them, as they both came from a nursery school and child development background. Later in life, Mary described Emma Plank as the "Godmother of Child Life." [27] She considered Emma Plank and B.J. Seabury as her mentors, and saw B.J. as a fellow advocate for child life in its struggle for professional recognition. When asked about her greatest accomplishments, Mary wrote that she was most proud of being a "midwife" at the birth of the Association for the Care of Children in Hospitals (ACCH) and of teaching the many young child life specialists who began their careers at CHOP. Mary was one of the founding members of ACCH in 1965. She attended the historical meeting at T. Berry Brazelton's home in Cape Cod. In the years to come, Mary served as the historian for the ACCH, as a member of the Editorial Advisory Board for Children's Health Care, Journal of the Association for the Care of Children's Health, and as chairwoman of the ACCH International Conference in 1967. She was elected by acclamation to a lifetime honorary member of the Child Life Council in 1983 and received the Child Life Council Distinguished Service Award in 1988. Mary wrote, "Our future as ACCH and CLC is onward and upward so far as I can see." [28]

ENDNOTES

1 Mary M. Brooks, Play for the Hospitalized Child, *Young Children, 24*(4), (1969): 219.
2 Mary M. Brooks, DVD, (Utica, NY: Utica College, Child Life Council Archives).
3 Brooks, Play for the Hospitalized Child.
4 Mary Brooks, Letter, (Utica, NY: Utica College, Child Life Council Archives, May 6, 1988).
5 Ibid.
6 Mabel Binner, They Play with You Here, *Modern Hospital, 44*(2), (1935): 54-58.
7 Dane G. Prugh, Elizabeth M. Staub, Harriet H. Sands, Ruth M. Kirschbaum, and Ellenora
   A. Lenihan, A Study of the Emotional Reactions of Children and Families to Hospitalization and Illness, *The American Journal of Orthopsychiatry, 23*(1), (1953): 70-106.
8 Luci Weber, phone conversation, February 20, 2013.
9 Brooks, DVD.
10 Nancy Burden, Play Ladies Help Sick Children, *The Sunday Bulletin, Philadelphia*,
   (March 2, 1969): 3.
11 Ibid.
12 Ibid.
13 *The Philadelphia Inquirer Magazine*, (September 11, 1966): 17.
14 Brooks, Play for the Hospitalized Child.
15 Ibid.
16 Eleanor Landsman, The Function of a Play Program in Pediatrics, *Children in Hospital
   Pediatric Annals*, (December 1972): 69.
17 Mary M. Brooks, Why Play in the Hospital? *Nursing Clinics of North America, 5*(3),
   (September 1970): 431.

18 Brooks, Play for the Hospitalized Child.

19 Ibid.

20 Pat Azarnoff and Sharon Flegal, A Pediatric Play Program, (Springfield, IL: Charles C. Thomas, 1975), 90.

21 Brooks, Play for the Hospitalized Child.

22 Brooks, Why Play in the Hospital?, 437.

23 Mary M. Brooks, Programmed Play Complements Care, *Hospitals*, *47*, (August 1, 1973): 87.

24 Mary M. Brooks, When a Young Child Must Be Hospitalized, *Health Education*, (May/June 1976): 22.

25 Mary M. Brooks, The Growth and Development of the Association for the Care of Children in Hospitals, *Journal of the Association for the Care of Children in Hospitals*, 4(1), (1975): 1-4.

26 Ibid.

27 Mary Brooks, Note, (Utica, NY: Utica College, Child Life Council Archives, May 5, 1993).

28 Mary Brooks, Letter, (Utica, NY: Utica College, Child Life Council Archives, May 6, 1988).

BIBLIOGRAPHY

Azarnoff, Pat, & Flegal, Sharon. *A Pediatric Play Program.* Springfield, IL: Charles C. Thomas, 1975/1990.

Binner, Mabel. They Play with You Here. *Modern Hospital, 44*(2), (1935): 54-58.

Brooks, Mary. Handwritten note. Utica, NY: Utica College, Child Life Council Archives, May 5, 1993.

Brooks, Mary M. Oral History (video recording). Utica, NY: Utica College, Child Life Council Archives, n.d.

Brooks, Mary M. Play for the Hospitalized Child. *Young Children, 24*(4), (1969): 219-224.

Brooks, Mary M. Why Play in the Hospital? *Nursing Clinics of North America, 5*(3), (1970): 431-441.

Brooks, Mary M. When a Young Child Must Be Hospitalized. *Health Education*, (May/June 1976): 22-24.

Brooks, Mary M. Handwritten letter. Utica, NY: Utica College, Child Life Council Archives, May 6, 1988.

Brooks, Mary McCleod. Programmed Play Complements Care. *Hospitals, 47*, (August 1, 1973): 78, 87.

Brooks, Mary McLeod. The Growth and Development of the Association for the Care of Children in Hospitals. *Journal of the Association for the Care of Children in Hospitals, 4*(1), (1975): 1-4.

Burden, Nancy. Play Ladies Help Sick Children. *The Sunday Bulletin, Philadelphia*, (March 2, 1969): 3.

Landsman, Eleanor. The Function of a Play Program in Pediatrics. *Children in Hospital Pediatric Annals*, (December 1972): 69.

n.a. Toy Time. *The Philadelphia Inquirer Magazine*, (September 11, 1966).

Prugh, Dane G., Staub, Elizabeth M., Sands, Harriet H., Kirschbaum, Ruth M., & Lenihan, Ellenora A. A Study of the Emotional Reactions of Children and Families to Hospitalization and Illness. *The American Journal of Orthopsychiatry, 23*(1), (1953): 70-106.

Weber, Luci. Phone conversation with Civita Brown, February 20, 2013. Luci Weber, CCLS, Retired Director of Child Life, Music Therapy & Patient Academics, All Children's Hospital, St. Petersburg, FL

CHAPTER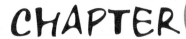

Emma Nuschi Plank (1905–1990): A Pioneer's Journey and Her Moral Compass

Stefi Rubin, *Wheelock College*

Prologue

In her preface to *On Development and Education of Young Children*, a selection of Lili Peller's papers she edited, Emma Nuschi Plank wrote that she hoped the book would "enrich the thinking of those who try to give stability to children in this troubled world."[1] In this readership, Plank included social workers, nurses and child development specialists, students in psychology and psychiatry, and "all those who have power to plan for children and stand for their rights and opportunities."[2] The hope that Plank expressed in regard to Peller's work also helps us understand the real-life achievements of Plank herself. She enriched the thinking and changed the practices of those who devoted their lives to helping children in need. From pre-WWII Vienna to the San Francisco Bay area in the 1940s, to three decades in Cleveland from the 1950s onward, until her death in Vienna in 1990, Plank's mission was to help children and to teach and support those who shared that commitment with her. This purpose served as Plank's moral compass. It guided her through genocidal threats under the Third Reich, through the uprooting from her native land, and through the significant hardships of reestablishing herself in mid-20th-century America. On this journey, Plank's values and commitments centered her. She helped transform the way we imagine and implement healthcare for children and families, a transformation that became most visible in the creation—in concert with her counterparts across the United States and Canada—of "child life" as a profession.

The creation of child life as a profession, however, is only part of the story of Emma Plank's contributions. In 1992, when I finished writing "What's In a Name: Child Life and the Play Lady Legacy," I knew almost instantly that there was more to tell about this remarkable woman.[3] The most fundamental and enduring dimension of her life that has yet to be fully told is the way in which her work was shaped by historical forces (including the places where she lived), and the vital and dynamic relations she maintained with a variety of like-minded, innovative thinkers and practitioners. This essay explores how her accomplishments were shaped both by their historical context and her collaborations with colleagues and friends.

Her Life in Europe

The older of two children born to Doris and Emil Spira, Emma Spira grew up in Vienna. Her life was profoundly affected by both world wars. At the end of WWI, the population of Vienna was decimated. As Plank later recalled in her typically understated tone, "It was a very trying time for mothers."[4] In 1918, her mother and her father, a civil servant, sent their 13-year-old daughter to her first group experience, a summer camp, which was for her "a milestone in my development."[5] This was likely the legendary camp organized by Eugenia Schwarzwald, a charismatic Viennese educator and social worker.[6] The next year, her parents made a major decision to send 14-year-old Nuschi to attend school in Sweden, a neutral country and one that could provide enough food, in contrast to postwar Austria.[7] Upon returning home, she felt that "school seemed so empty."[8] Learning a foreign language and living in another country at a young age gave her a broader perspective about history. She thought that if "the older generation had gotten us into this mess, we, the younger generation would lead us out of it. We were optimistic enough to think that what we did mattered."[9] She added that when she came back from Sweden, "I had seen what a country *without war* was like. I was determined…that I wanted to be an educator!"[10] The next summer, she proceeded to co-lead a summer camp for 40 children in a castle ruin in the Dolomites, thus beginning her work with children.

By the time Plank was 16, she'd heard about the Montessori School directed by Lili Peller. Only 23 herself, Peller had studied for 2 years with Montessori in London, and returned to Vienna to found the "Haus der Kinder" (The Children's House). She also established an apprenticeship program consisting of five girls, ages 16 to 18. Nuschi was one of those five girls, all of whom lived at the school where they worked. As Plank recalled years later, they were "full of hopes for the young republic," even if the school was located in "one of the drabbest working class districts of the city impoverished by World War I."[11] With limited funding, the school expected the girls first to serve what was called "a year of practice." For Plank, this meant kitchen work, in exchange for invaluable training as a Montessori teacher. And she enjoyed the fact that the children, too, were kitchen helpers, with child-size tables and sinks.[12] From the beginning, in other words, the work was done with devotion. Plank wrote in her preface to Peller's papers that the apprentices "were devoted to a purpose." That purpose was to provide "services to underprivileged children."[13] The dedicated way the apprentices lived and worked, she said many years later, reminded her of Peace Corps workers in that they were imbued with a hope "that what we did really mattered and should help build a better world."[14]

The Vienna Montessori School became a training site for many educators and social workers from all over central Europe. Plank recalled that students could enroll in a 2-year course, "culminating with four months of study with Montessori herself."[15] Eric Erikson, for instance, enrolled in the program.[16] After two years as an apprentice, Plank advanced herself by learning Italian to understand lectures by Montessori, whom Plank said visited the school "repeatedly and was deeply interested in our program."[17] By 1926, Plank had earned a certificate in kindergarten and elementary education from the Teacher's College and a year later, a diploma from the International Montessori Training Course in Berlin. By 1931, Nuschi herself was selected as the director of the Haus der Kinder. Two years later, her mentor, Peller, married and moved to Israel and then on to the United States in 1937, where she worked as a psychoanalyst in New York. When she died in 1966, Plank spoke at a commemorative service at the Waldorf-Astoria Hotel and secured Peller's place as an intellectual and early childhood educator by editing *Lili E. Peller, On Development and Education of Young Children*, a collection of 19 of her papers spanning 40 years.[18]

Vienna in the 1920s and 1930s was intellectually alive with new theories about human development, with psychoanalysis one of the most lively of those currents. Plank credited Peller with having the vision to enable Montessori teachers to attend biweekly seminars with Anna Freud.[19] In these seminars, Plank noted, "psychoanalysis and its meaning for educators and education opened up for us."[20] She explained, "We trained not as child therapists, but as psychoanalytically oriented educators."[21] Plank completed advanced training for teachers at the Vienna Psychoanalytic Institute from 1935–1938. This is one of the best examples of the rich intellectual cross-fertilization that Plank encountered in Vienna.

Surviving the Anschluss, three days of terror in March 1938 (when Germany annexed Austria into the Third Reich), Nuschi and her husband, Robert, a lawyer, had to escape. They would have to go through the difficult and frightening process of acquiring the necessary emigration papers, including affidavits and sponsorship letters.[22] British immigration officials accepted them, but only on the condition that they could prove that their ultimate destination was the United States. Serendipitously, their sponsors were two sisters, one a psychologist in New York, the other a social worker living in San Francisco, who had earlier visited the Vienna Montessori School.[23] When the Planks first arrived in London, en route to California, they were asked to direct a Basque Children's Home, where 30 refugee children were living. These children had survived Franco's bombings and thus, like the Planks, had been uprooted by war and the violent rise of Fascism in Europe.

Crisscrossing America

The Planks crossed the Atlantic on a Dutch ship that docked in New York. When she next arrived as a total stranger in San Francisco, Plank taught in and eventually directed the progressive and highly regarded Presidio Hill School. How did this happen? Part of the answer is in her connection to Josephine Whitney Duveneck, daughter of a prominent Boston family. The Duveneck's were philanthropic activists in the Bay area. She and her husband had sheltered European refugees at their Hidden Villa ranch, and they had assisted Japanese-American families dealing with interment.[24] Josephine was also a former director of the Presidio Hill School, where Dewey's ideas about creative expression and learning by doing were core values.[25] Dewey's commitment to social justice also informed the school's central values and made it a place where "European refugees could get help in their transition to American life."[26] At first, however, Nuschi found work as an attendant in an orphanage in Oakland, California, and it was there that she first met Duveneck. In *Living On Two Levels,* her autobiography, Josephine recalls "Someone introduced her to me....and I was fascinated by her description of the school she had conducted in Austria."[27] Duveneck was familiar with Montessori preschool educational materials, but she apparently learned from Plank about the materials used in elementary classrooms. More significantly, however, was that Emma Plank herself impressed Duveneck, who wrote, referring to the Planks, "There were many memorable incidents in finding jobs for uprooted people.... Some very dear friendships evolved from those emergencies, and several have lasted our lives."[28] Duvenick quickly sized up Nuschi's situation. Duveneck added, "It seemed to me preposterous that a woman of her dynamic personality and achievement should be making beds and scrubbing pots and pans. Although her English was pretty scant, I persuaded her to talk to a group of teachers and show her educational materials. Then I offered her a teaching job at Presidio Hill School, where she later became principal."[29]

When forced to leave behind her school and its students, Emma Plank nevertheless took with her Montessori materials, as if she was equipping herself for a future that might build upon her past. What hopes did she bring with her as she hurriedly packed a trunk for her journey to the United States? How is it that Josephine's path crossed with hers in such a surprising, transformative way? Whatever the case was, they had a profound meeting of minds and values, so much so that when Nuschi became a U.S. citizen, Josephine gave her a treasured gift of Walt Whitman's book of poetry, as if to say, "Welcome, fellow American!"[30]

While directing Presidio Hill, Plank attended Mills College and completed her master's degree in child development in 1947. She then returned to Vienna for 2 years (1948-1950) to serve as a special projects director for the American Friends Service Committee, where she developed courses for the Pedagogic Institute and the Vienna School of Social Work. Recognized for her contributions to the well-being of children, she was awarded the Medal of the City of Vienna in 1949. Concurrently, Robert was drafted into the army and fought in the Battle of the Bulge.[31] As a veteran, he then started over professionally, earning a master's degree in social work from UCLA Berkeley in 1948 and working in that field for the Veteran's Administration. He also wrote social commentary and science fiction, including a book analyzing George Orwell's *1984*.[32]

The Cleveland Years

After living in San Francisco for almost 10 years, why then did the Planks uproot themselves a second time and move to Cleveland? In a videotaped interview, Nuschi reminisced about how happy she and Robert had been in San Francisco and yet how compelling was the invitation from Dr. Anny Katan to come to work at the Children's House of University Hospital in Cleveland. This preschool for children with emotional and behavioral problems—later renamed the Hanna Perkins School—pioneered the use of psychoanalysis with young children and parent involvement in treatment.[33] After two more letters from Katan (whose child had attended the Montessori School in Vienna), the Planks decided to accept the offer and move to Ohio in 1950.[34] Nuschi became the school's administrative director.

Dr. Katan, herself a Viennese child psychoanalyst, came to Cleveland in 1946 at the recommendation of Anna Freud, her teacher, and Dr. Douglas Bond, the director of psychiatry at University Hospital, a key figure in the psychoanalytic community of Cleveland.

Dr. Frederick Robbins also moved to Cleveland in 1952 and would in 1954 become one of three co-recipients of the Nobel Prize in physiology or medicine for their work on the polio virus. Appointed professor of pediatrics in the medical school of Western Reserve University, Dr. Robbins also became the director of the Department of Pediatrics and Contagious Diseases at Cleveland Metropolitan General Hospital (later renamed Metrohealth Medical Center). Many of the pediatric patients, especially those with tuberculosis, were hospitalized for long periods on dreary wards. Dr. Robbins asked his new colleagues whom they could recommend to help make the pediatric wards more child-friendly. Dr. Bond knew of Nuschi through the Hanna Perkins School and urged Dr. Robbins to contact her. Nuschi visited the pediatric unit and thought she could be of help. Robbins asked her to write a foundation grant in order to fund the pilot program in its first 2 years, after which it was funded by the hospital.[35] By 1955, Nuschi had founded the hospital's Child Life and Education Program. She had in the process involved graduate students in the program's development, and she would later say that one of her dreams was to have every medical student spend time in a child life program in order to learn first how children develop, and later learn how they are affected by and cope with illness and hospitalization.[36]

After 7 years of directing the program, Nuschi published *Working with Children in Hospitals: A Guide for the Professional Team*. Filled with black-and-white photos of playroom and bedside activities, children's artwork, and an illustrated medical preparation story, the book became a classic, going into a second printing, revised and expanded, in 1971, and eventually translated into German, Spanish, French, and Japanese. The book's cover page indicates the book was written "with the assistance of Marlene A. Ritchie," Plank's first assistant, a teacher and nursing instructor. The second edition contained a new dedication, "to the memory of Lili E. Peller and Annie Reich, M.D."[37]

In his forward to the first edition, Dr. Robbins emphasized how the world of pediatrics has undergone remarkable changes, especially the specialization of doctors and the shortage of nurses. He voiced great concern that "hospital experiences risked becoming too impersonal…with a great deal of attention being paid to the child's illness and too little to his feelings." He also said that a "perceptive colleague" of his had often said, "Someone must defend the child against the system."

It's easy to imagine that the colleague he is referring to was Emma Plank. He goes on to write that "it is as the child's advocate against the system that the child-care worker fulfills her most important role."[38] Within the book itself, essentially the first textbook in the field of child life, Nuschi asks, "What is the child care worker we have just mentioned? What does she do?" Plank answers her questions by reciting possible titles: "Neither teacher nor play lady nor play therapist quite captures what they actually do."[39] She goes on to clarify that the childcare worker is a person "on the clinical team who is responsible for the children at play and at meal times, or in the hospital school, but is not involved in the nursing function as such, though she may help prepare children for medical procedures or surgery through such activities as dramatic play or earnest and factual conversation in the playroom."[40]

During the 1960s, Plank maintained a dual focus, locally and nationally. Locally, she fostered interdisciplinary teamwork. She also extended the scope of her department by expanding a busy outpatient clinic and an innovative service called Play Corner, for children who are "not sick themselves but whose mothers are clinic patients, or whose mothers are visiting siblings or other family members in the hospital."[41]

Nationally, she assumed numerous leadership roles and served as a model of energetic engagement. She kept her early childhood ties active, while simultaneously developing the hospital program; for example, she was elected president of the Midwestern Association for Nursery Education (1961–1962). In 1965 she was identified as one of six founders of the Association for the Care of Children in Hospitals and went on to serve as its president (1968–1970). In 1970, she was a delegate to the White House Conference on Children and she participated in a symposium, "The Effects of Hospitalization on Children," sponsored by the Extension Division of the San Francisco Psychoanalytic Society. She was invited to the latter by Evelyn Oremland, the Mills College professor who later founded that college's child life program.[42] That same year, Plank was awarded the Gold Medal from the Montessori Centennial. When she retired at age 66 in 1971, she had achieved the rank professor emeritus of child development at Case Western Reserve University.

Almost a decade later, Nuschi witnessed the establishment of the Child Life Council, the organizational home for this emerging profession. When Robert died in 1983, she returned to Vienna for her remaining years. She posthumously edited her husband's book on Orwell.[43] Wheelock College in Boston awarded her an honorary doctorate in 1988, as part of its centennial and in recognition of her influence on its own child life department and its "Hospitalized Child in London" program. Two years later, she died in Vienna and was buried with her husband. In 1995, ACCH, the organization she was instrumental in forming, held a featured symposium on her life and work at its 30th Conference in Boston. In 2005, at the 50th anniversary of the founding of the Child Life and Education program at Metrohealth Medical Center, a panel presentation honored Plank at the Child Life Council Conference in Nashville, Tennessee, and displayed a reprint of her book, which had gone out of print. And, in her memory, the Child Life Council's Annual Conference begins each year with the "Emma Plank Keynote Address."

Emma Plank's life and work represent the integration of child development and psychoanalytic theories with the educational theories of Dewey and Montessori. She aimed to unite play and education in conceptualizing the roles of childcare workers. Furthermore, she was known to be always on the go and warmly interacting with patients, families, staff, and students. In their chapter entitled "Advocates and Ombudsmen," Hardgrove and Dawson wrote that Plank was to become "one of the best-known pioneers in the ombudsman role."[44] In their observational research, they found her to be constantly visiting units, interacting one on one and in groups with children, staff, and parents. They witnessed how "she carries out a complex job on many levels and supervises her staff as well as students in training."[45] Hardgove admired how much Plank "sees each child in a personal and individual way."[46] She also reached out to the community as a liaison, consultant, and teacher. Hardgrove learned that she "goes into the community to talk with college students or to parents' groups about the emotional needs of sick children, about preparing children for the hospital, and about the ways hospitalization can enhance growth."[47]

In addition to her direct clinical and administrative roles, Plank was a scholar as well as an advocate. Starting in 1951 as an instructor in child development at Western Reserve University, she had within 20 years risen to the rank of professor emeritus. She had published over 30 journal articles, many of which reflected her interdisciplinary expertise. These journals include *The Journal of Nursery Education, Social Casework,* and *Pediatrics.*

When the War on Poverty and the civil rights movement stirred the nation to action in the 1960s, Plank, an advocate for the well-being of all children, recognized that the hospital population was a microcosm of the larger society. The photographs in her 1962 book show both African American and Caucasian children in the hospital's patient population. At the symposium held in San Francisco in 1970, she pointed out that integration fostered a positive climate for both children and parents.[48] She explained, "We have seen the remarkable ability of people to change their opinions on racial integration through their hospital experiences. These unexpected and often first contacts as equals between children and parents of different races have brought rewards. Firm bonds, through their common destiny as patients, have developed between some children, and were strengthened through the good feelings among the interracial staff."[49]

Conclusion

Emma Plank's life story was informed by questions of social injustice and her efforts to address them. Her life and work are testimony to her determination "to plan for children and stand for their rights and opportunities."[50] Hundreds of children, parents, and colleagues benefited from her intelligence and compassion. Renowned as the "mother" of child life, she had a confident yet unassuming manner that was grounded in her steadfast core values.

In 1992, Vienna University Hospital invited Evelyn Oremland to give a talk about her mentor and friend's original contributions to pediatric care.[51] Years earlier, her husband, Dr. Jerome Oremland, a friend and psychiatrist, had written that Plank's efforts aimed to ameliorate the suffering of sick children and to decrease their fears "by helping them understand what is happening to them and what they are experiencing."[52] From an early age, Emma Plank had an inventive, independent mind of her own. She also had a strong moral compass, based on her deep understanding of the needs of children and their parents. Her values, along with her interpersonal skills, have inspired others to join together on the ward, or in a classroom, or community center to stand with her on behalf of children's rights and opportunities. Their work is her most enduring legacy.

ENDNOTES

1 Lili E Peller, *On Development and Education of Young Children, Selected Papers*, ed. by Emma N. Plank, (New York: Philosophical Library Inc., 1978), xxii.
2 Ibid.
3 Stefi Rubin, What's in a Name? Child Life and the Play Lady Legacy, *Children's Health Care, 21*, (Winter 1992): 4-13.
4 *Emma Plank and Child Health Care: An Innovator's Journey.* Carlyn Yanda interviews Emma Plank, (Cleveland, OH: Educational Media Dept., Case Western Reserve University, 1984), VHS videotape.

5 Yanda, *Emma Plank and Child Health Care.*

6 Elena Shapira, s.v. Eugenie Schwarzwald, *Jewish Women: A Comprehensive Historical Encyclopedia,* (Jewish Women's Archive, March 1, 2009), accessed November 17, 2013, http://jwa.org/encyclopedia/article/schwarzwald-eugenie.

7 Yanda, *Emma Plank and Child Health Care.*

8 Ibid.

9 Ibid.

10 Ibid.

11 Peller, *On Development,* xv.

12 Yanda, *Emma Plank and Child Health Care.*

13 Peller, *On Development,* xvi.

14 Ibid.

15 Ibid., xvii.

16 Ibid.

17 Ibid.

18 *Montessori-Zentrum,* Wien, 2004. Lili Peller-Roubiczek-die "grande dame" der Wiener Montessori-Bewegung der Zwischenkriegszeit. Mag.a Jutta Haslinger-Mayer. (Lili Peller Roubiczek-the "grande dame"of the Vienna Montessori Movement in the interwar period) http://montessori.at/home/publicationen/publikationen5.xhtml.

19 Peller, *On Development,* x.

20 Ibid., xviii.

21 Ibid.

22 Yanda, *Emma Plank and Child Health Care.*

23 Ibid.

24 www.hiddenvilla.org/about

25 www.presdiohill.org/about

26 Ibid.

27 Josephine Duveneck, *Living on Two Levels, An Autobiography* (Los Altos, CA: William Kaufmann, Inc.,1978), 228.

28 Ibid.

29 Ibid.

30 Yanda, *Emma Plank and Child Health Care.*

31 Ibid.

32 Robert Plank, *George Orwell's Guide Through Hell, A Psychological Study of* 1984. (Holicong, PA: The Borgo Press, 1986).

33 Encyclopedia of Cleveland History, s.v. "Hanna Perkins School," http://ech.case.edu/cgi/article.pl?id=HPS, last modified July 7, 1997

34 Yanda, *Emma Plank and Child Health Care.*

35 Ibid.

36 *Emma Plank Tribute: Celebrating 50 Years Of Child Life,* (Cleveland, OH: Metrohealth Medical Center, 2005), DVD.

37 Emma Plank, *Working with Children in Hospitals, A Guide for the Professional Team,* (Cleveland: The Press of Case Western Reserve, 1971).

38 Plank, *Working with Children in Hospitals*, 1962, x.

39 Plank, *Working with Children in Hospitals*, 1971, 7.

40 Ibid.

41 E. Oremland and J. Oremland, *The Effects of Hospitalization On Children, Models for Their Care*, (Springfield, IL: Charles C. Thomas Publisher, 1973), 33.

42 E. Oremland, *Protecting the Emotional Development of the Ill Child: The Essence of the Child Life Profession*, (Madison, CT: Psychosocial Press, 2000), x.

43 Robert Plank, *George Orwell's Guide Through Hell, A Psychological Study of 1984* (2nd ed.), (Holicong, PA: The Borgo Press, 1994).

44 C. Hardgrove and R. Dawson, *Parents and Children in the Hospital, The Family's Role in Pediatrics*, (Boston: Little Brown Company, 1972), 109.

45 Ibid.

46 Ibid.

47 Hardgrove and Dawson, 117.

48 Oremland and Oremland, *The Effects of Hospitalization on Children*, 247.

49 Ibid., 247-248.

50 Emma Plank, *Working with Children in Hospitals, A Guide for the Professional Team*. xxii.

51 Oremland, *Protecting the Emotional Development of the Ill Child*, 239.

52 Oremland and Oremland, *The Effects of Hospitalization on Children*, 331.

BIBLIOGRAPHY

Bourke, Eoin. *The Austrian Anschluss in History and Literature*. Galway, Ireland: Arlen House, 2000.

Brazelton, T. Berry. *Learning to Listen, a Life Caring for Children*. Philadelphia: Da Capa Press, 2013.

Duveneck, Josephine Whitney. *Life on Two Levels: An Autobiography*. Los Altos, CA: William Kaufmann Inc., 1978.

Emma Plank and Child Health Care: An Innovator's Journey. Carlyn Yanda interviews Emma Plank. Cleveland, OH: Educational Media Department, Case Western Reserve University, 1984. VHS videotape, 41 minutes.

Friedman, Lawrence. *Identity's Architect, A Biography of Erik H. Erikson*. New York: Scribner, 1999.

Gamble, Vanessa. *Making a Place for Ourselves: The Black Hospital Movement 1920-1945*. New York: Oxford University Press, 1995.

Hardgrove, Carol, & Dawson, Rosemary B. *Parents and Children in the Hospital, the Family's Role in Pediatrics*. Boston: Little Brown Company, 1972.

Kramer, Rita. *Maria Montessori, a Biography*. Reading, MA: Addison-Wesley Publishing Co., 1976.

Legarreta, Dorothy. *The Guernica Generation: Basque Refugee Children of the Spanish Civil War*. Reno: University of Nevada Press, 1984.

Oremland, Evelyn. Edited by Jerome D. Oremland. *Protecting the Emotional Development of the Ill Child, the Essence of the Child Life Profession*. Madison, CT: Psychosocial Press, 2000.

Oremland, Evelyn, & Oremland, Jerome, eds. *The Effects of Hospitalization on Children, Models for Their Care.* Springfield, IL: Charles C. Thomas Publisher, 1973.

Peller, Lili E. Edited by Emma N. Plank. *On Development and Education of Young Children, Selected Papers.* New York: Philosophical Library, 1978.

Plank, Emma N., with the assistance of Marlene A. Ritchie. *Working with Children in Hospitals, a Guide for the Professional Team.* Cleveland: The Press of Case Western Reserve University, 1962.

Plank, Emma N., with the assistance of Marlene A. Ritchie. *Working with Children in Hospitals, a Guide for the Professional Team* (2nd ed., rev. and expanded). Cleveland: The Press of Case Western Reserve University, 1971.

Plank, Emma N., with the assistance of Marlene A. Ritchie. *Working with Children in Hospitals, a Guide for the Professional Team* (3rd ed.). Cleveland: Metrohealth Medical Center, 2005.

Plank, Robert. *George Orwell's Guide Through Hell, A Psychological Study of 1984.* Holicong, PA: The Borgo Press, 1986, 1994.

Rubin, Stefi. What's in a Name? Child Life and the Play Lady Legacy. *Children's Health Care, 21,* (1992): 4-13.

Thompson, Richard, ed. *The Handbook of Child Life, a Guide for Pediatric Psychosocial Care.* Springfield, IL: Charles C. Thomas, 2009.

Young-Bruehl, Elizabeth. *Anna Freud, a Biography.* New York: Summit, 1988.

CHAPTER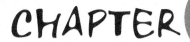

A New Era: From Play Activities to Child Life at Johns Hopkins

Jerriann Myers Wilson, *The Johns Hopkins Children's Hospital (Retired)*

"I'm just not 'on fire' to teach," I told Dorothy Arnold, the director of vocational guidance at Baltimore's Goucher College, in 1962, with only a few months left before I was to graduate. I had majored in education and child development, student-taught in a first-grade classroom, and interviewed for teaching positions on the East Coast but I did not feel like I was taking the right direction for me. To her question of what I wanted to do, I assured her I wanted to work with children—yes, maybe even in a hospital. I was aware of nursing and occupational therapy and knew I wasn't prepared for those professions. She mentioned that Johns Hopkins Hospital had a program called "Child Life" and that I should explore it. I telephoned the program with all of the enthusiasm of someone who thought she had "invented a new job," interviewed, received a job offer, and began in August 1962 never having had a practicum, an internship, or even a personal hospital experience as a child. But, what was the origin of this program that I had never heard of?

The Developing Play Activities Program

The birth of the Hopkins's play program began with two visionaries: Onica Prall and Helen Schnetzer, women who like Anne Smith had the skills and the wherewithal to make a difference in the lives of hospitalized children.[1] Prall, a child development professor and founder of the Lab School at Hood College in Frederick, Maryland (1929–1969), contacted Johns Hopkins Hospital early in 1943 to volunteer her services during the summer as a contribution to the war effort because there was such a shortage of personnel, especially nurses.[2]   Prall asked only for room and board if they could use her services. She was referred to Helen Schnetzer, then nursing supervisor of pediatrics in the Harriet Lane Home for Invalid Children at Hopkins. Schnetzer enthusiastically accepted Prall's offer. Prall described Schnetzer and her goals:

> She was a brilliant young woman, full of all kinds of creative ideas. One, she pushed hard—namely that student nurses should know something about the development of normal children and that someone other than a nurse should teach them. Secondly, a person should be procured to direct play activities for the hospitalized children—again a non hospital-oriented person.[3]

Prall met with Schnetzer at the hospital and agreed to work with the children and to teach development courses to both the student nurses and the graduate nurses.

Prall spent only 9 weeks in the Harriet Lane Home that summer but during that period she had a positive feeling about how she was received by the medical staff. She recalled the early days:

> After the first few weeks of the program the few skeptics were won over. Dr. Edwards Park, Chief of Pediatrics, was from the beginning whole-heartedly behind the project and often called me to go on the weekly rounds so that his   interns could understand the value of the program. Soon they and the residents started putting suggestions in the Order book for me.[4]

In addition to teaching a series of 10 two-hour classes for the nurses and the nursing students, Prall enlisted six volunteer student interns to work with her—five child development students and one pre-med student. They each worked five half-days a week in the playroom or at bedside, offering table games, block play, reading, and craft activities. Prall filled the role of "Play Teacher" and worked seven days a week. She instituted group play and group meal times in the playroom. Prall described a positive response from children, parents, and staff.[5] Members of the Auxiliary Board commented that they did not hear any crying; and that parents seemed relieved their children were less apprehensive.[6]   Prall noted that the playroom was messier than usual but that children seemed more at ease. Schnetzer was pleased with Prall's accomplishments.

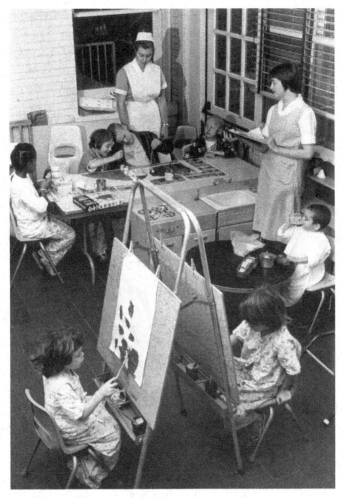

Early activities at The Johns Hopkins Hospital playroom: painting and games
The Alan Mason Chesney Medical Archives of The Johns Hopkins Medical Institutions. Used by Permission Permit 14970

The Hopkins administration decided in midsummer that they would like to make this program permanent and offered Prall the position. Because of her commitment to Hood, she declined, but offered to find a candidate from the next year's graduating class, which she did. In September 1944, the Pediatric Nursing Department established Play Activities as one of its services and hired Mary Caulkins Johnson, a new Hood child development graduate, to fill the first position.[7] Johnson and future staff were funded for the next two decades by the Hospital Women's Board and all were employees of the Johns Hopkins Nursing School. The play teachers continued to carry dual roles of providing a program for the children and families as well as instructing student nurses about playroom activities to add to their understanding of child development. The supervision of student nurses by the play teacher staff in the playrooms was an important part of pediatric nursing education. In the *Hopkins Alumnae Magazine*, one student nurse shared her impressions:

> Play School...helps to distribute the service of one Play Director to a group   of one hundred or more children in four or five geographical locations and...it is an effort to meet an educational need in the nurse who must work with children.[8]

In the intervening years, several dozen women with a background in child development were hired and the staff size grew to number five or six. Prall continued to serve as a consultant to the program for several years, providing the program with child development student interns from Hood College until she retired in 1969.

New Attitudes in Child Care

Backing up a little, it is interesting to reflect on the Hopkins Play Activities program within the context of the 1940s through the 1960s when issues of importance to healthcare personnel and to parents were undergoing change. In 1937, H.L. Mencken, journalist at the Baltimore Sun in a series about The Johns Hopkins Hospital for the Baltimore Sun, described the need for children over 2 years of age to be entertained with toys. He commented on the parents' role:

> The children make good patients, and after the first few days seldom cry for their mothers. But when they see their mothers again, they begin crying again, so visiting is not encouraged. In fact, Sunday is the only regular visiting day. But when a child is desperately ill, of course, its mother may come at any time, and stay all night. For fear that they may bring in infections, mothers are seldom permitted to enter the wards. Instead their children, lying in cribs, are wheeled out to them.[9]

From the physician point of view, for instance, U.S. Surgeon General C. Everett Koop reminded us that children were treated physically as small adults as late as the 1940s and that children died in surgery because of errors in medications.[10] It is well known that children also were regarded emotionally as small adults. However, in 1965, Dr. Edward Mason of Harvard summarized a variety of research studies undertaken from the 1920s through the 1950s which focused attention on the emotional needs of hospitalized children including preparation, need for activities, parental presence, and more.[11] A change was coming.

In addition to the shifting perspectives of physicians, the nursing profession was also moving forward in attending to the needs of children and their families. A growing influence on pediatric care came from the nursing profession as they reexamined their training methods for nursing education. Cindy Connolly, Yale University School of Nursing, in an article reviewing the early professionalization of pediatric nursing, summarized:

> In addition to the attention paid to the infectious diseases, the late nineteenth and early twentieth century nursing literature also emphasized the unique age-related considerations of child health care. Though pediatric nurses did not use growth and development-related terminology in the same way we do to-day, their ideas were nonetheless creative and demonstrated the practical utility underpinning the new field of psychology…in ways that acknowledged the cognitive and physical differences between children and adults.[12]

By 1940, a major goal for Anna D. Wolf, director of nursing at Hopkins, was to "upgrade nursing-education programs."[13] She had observed that nursing students were given extensive ward service but little educational subject matter related to the needs of convalescing children. Therefore, as was the case for Anne Smith at Chicago Memorial Children's Hospital, the time was right for the collaboration of nursing and child development experts. The meeting of Helen Schnetzer and Onica Prall resulted in changes in attitudes and practices toward children and families, eventually leading to what I might have called, "the invention of a new job."

A New Era: Child Life

The focus beyond the medical needs of the child, to now include a more holistic view of the child, was beginning to emerge and was reflected early at Johns Hopkins as the play activities program developed further. In 1961, Robert Dombro was hired, having previously worked with children with hearing impairments. At the suggestion of Dr. Robert E. Cooke, chairman of pediatrics, Dombro changed the name of the program from Play Activities to Child Life.[14] This was meant to signify the broader role of the program to include not only play activities, but also a variety of facets of a child's life in the hospital.[15] In a letter to Mary Murphy, Dombro described the following components of the newly envisioned Child Life Program:[16]

- Academic education is provided the hospitalized child.
- Meaningful play activities are conducted for [sic] the child.
- Rapport with parents is established to help them adjust more easily to the hospital environment.
- An education program is conducted for the student nurses that emphasizes the value of individual and group experiences.
- An outpatient department program is [being] established both for parents and their youngsters stressing the importance of leisure time activities and health education.
- A strong volunteer program is [being] developed so that more of the hospitalized children can receive services.
- Community agencies are being asked to participate both in the inpatient and outpatient areas in order to enrich our program and to establish good community relationships.

Dombro hired Barbara Schuyler Haas, formerly the director of a cooperative nursery school, as child life supervisor, to oversee the staff who worked with the patients—that is, four child life instructors and a teacher. The Harriet Lane Home building housed a ward medical unit, a private medical unit, an infant unit, and an outpatient area. Children with surgical diagnoses were admitted to a separate floor in the Halsted Surgical Building. Three instructors were responsible for the programming on the two medical units and the surgical unit. The fourth instructor supervised volunteers who provided day and evening programming for children.[17] Acknowledgment of the needs of hospitalized infants had yet to be incorporated into the programming at this point in time.

Students were continuing to play a role by providing needed services in the pediatric outpatient area. Two full-time positions were created for Antioch College students who came under a work-study arrangement for 3- or 6-month periods. The students provided play activities for outpatients as well as for pediatric patients who were admitted to adult areas. This student arrangement, similar to that described earlier by Anne Smith, was an important first step in the development of training programs for what we now commonly refer to as child life.[18]

This was a time of change because of the new leadership that Dombro and Haas brought to the program. In 1962, I was assigned to the ward medical unit as the child life instructor where my task was to present good play experiences—meaning that they were educational and therapeutic in nature. Play and school activities supported normal development and facilitated the expression of emotions. This provided continuity between home and hospital for each child and helped create a sense of normalcy, which was important for a child's adjustment to the setting. The children had many opportunities to choose from a variety of activities such as toys, games, books, a housekeeping corner, music, movies, and television. The atmosphere was permissive in order to allow the children a good deal of independence.

A school program on my unit was provided part of each day by the teacher who was responsible for the school program on the three inpatient units. She used a child's own schoolwork when available or introduced themes (travel, the sea, the farm) for group lessons to allow children to explore new ideas.[19] A child could be included in school without regard to length of stay. A large closet/storage area provided space for a library that was an important component of the educational program.

Child life instructors had what we called "therapeutic" conversations with the patients. This was before formal psychological preparation was considered as part of the child life program. Of interest to our staff at the time was the work of a new colleague, Clarissa Robins Hobbs, also employed in 1962, who had just completed her master's thesis, titled "A Comparison of the Play Material Preferences of Hospitalized and Non-Hospitalized Children," in which she found that the most preferred toys for the hospitalized children were medically related toys.[20] This was my early exposure to the study of hospitalized children and play. Although Emma Plank had published her remarkable book, *Working with Children in Hospitals*, in 1962, I was not aware of it. Somehow, a connection between the leaders at Johns Hopkins and other leading children's hospitals such as City Hospital, Cleveland (later The Children's Hospital at MetroHealth Medical Center) where Emma Plank was situated must have been occurring. However, as a novice during the early 1960s, I was not yet engaged in the happenings around what would soon emerge as the Association for the Care of Children in Hospitals. Plank's advocacy supporting the coordination of activities for children across disciplines was an important breakthrough for developing activity programs.

At Johns Hopkins this coordination was evident through the collaboration of nursing and child life. Building on the experience begun by Onica Prall, student nurses spent 2 weeks of their 16-week pediatric experience in the playroom using play and art activities with patients under the supervision of the child life instructor. This served as a laboratory for observation and was coupled with 20 hours of classes in child development. In addition to the daily conferences between the student nurses and the child life instructors, each student nurse presented a report comparing the needs of the hospitalized patient with those needs outside the hospital.[21] The nursing school catalogue described the value of student nurse participation in child life:

> Assignments…in the Child Life Program provide opportunities for the student to learn suitable guidance techniques and to develop the ability to make effective use of play to meet the child's interests and needs…the concepts of normal growth and development and their implications are presented as dynamic forces which affect the child physically, mentally, socially, and emotionally.[22]

Greater coordination occurred as pediatric services were merged under one roof. In 1964 the new Children's Medical and Surgical Center (CMSC, also referred to as the Children's Center) was completed and all pediatric services were finally together. The title of "child life instructor" became "child life teacher" (the "specialist" term would not be adopted by the Hopkins program until 1984). The expanded space and staff allowed for the enhancement of all child life programs. The foundation that would guide the child life efforts for the future had already been established in the Harriet Lane Home. Supported by Dr. Cooke, the Dombro-Haas philosophy acknowledged the effects of hospitalization and other healthcare experiences on children and their families and resolved to help ameliorate these effects through the child life program and its focus. By 1964, the goal was:

> …to have a permanent [Child Life] staff actively engaged in the day-to-day programming for patients. They will have concern both for the growth and developmental needs of the child and for the emotional aspects of the experiences that confront the child and his family…. Staff members recognize the potential adverse effects of illness and hospitalization on behavior of both children and their families but also believe that a hospital experience can be a strengthening one for the whole family.[23]

The 12-story Children's Center had child life coverage on four inpatient floors with units for chronically ill children, medical patients, surgical patients, and adolescents. Each of these floors had a very large "play-school-dining" area. Play has always been the basis for child life work and it was part of the daily program. Dombro stated that "a major concern of the Child Life Program Staff is the creation of a setting in which children feel free to explore, to investigate, to experiment, to choose activities, and to express themselves."[24] The medical and surgical units each cared for 36 patients and had two child life teachers. Each morning they divided the large rooms to create a space for preschool on one side and school on the other. Pediatric surgeon J. Alex Haller, Jr. once described hospitalization as an "adventure," to which pediatrician Henry Seidel added, "An educational experience provides a familiar foothold, a means for acting out his fears, a means for providing a secure base from which to explore and profit from this new adventure."[25]

Group mealtimes for lunch and dinner were provided in the playrooms as a part of the daily routine and were important as a way to provide elements of a normal environment. The child life teachers assisted children as they ate their meals and they appreciated the value of this experience; however, one teacher was taken aback ever so slightly when one child called out, "Waitress, I need a straw, please."

School activities were also offered on the adolescent unit and the unit for chronically ill children. Education was an important part of the daily program, another way to provide normalcy for children no matter what was their length of stay. A library and book cart service were established and run by volunteers for years until a professional librarian was hired. An outdoor play deck made open-air activities possible for the patients and families. Child life coverage was provided for the pediatric intensive care unit, the outpatient area, and the infant-toddler unit. No play area existed for infants when the CMSC opened but with input from child life and nursing, a play area was eventually built.

Visiting hours in the 1940s in the Harriet Lane Building were twice a week for 1 hour. These hours were expanded to 2 to 9 hours daily for family members, depending upon the unit. The pediatric surgery unit was the most restrictive. Parents were only allowed to "live-in" on the private floor as the large ward areas with two to four beds in each cubicle on the other floors did not accommodate parents. With the new facility, sleeping space for parents was provided with chair beds and visiting hours were expanded from morning until evening; 24-hour visiting came later. A need was recognized for a liaison person to work with parents and hospital staff. With Dombro in charge of developing the family liaison program, a liaison person trained in child development was seen as appropriate in the role. However, in time, the role required a nursing focus and the liaison role was transferred to the nursing department. Eventually the family liaison role would become the heart of the program for family-centered care.

Overall, all aspects of training provided by the child life program were enhanced.[26] There were teaching opportunities with residents in both pediatrics and pediatric surgery as well as with the fourth-year medical students. The student nurse program which had begun in the Harriet Lane Building was intensified. A pre-clinical course in human development was introduced and new courses in play, child development, and effects of illness and hospitalization were added to enable the student nurses to have a more successful 2-week child life training program. Eventually the internship was a strong part of the program; it was a 10-week experience offered three times a year with five to eight participants from colleges all over the country. Indeed, the profile of this new program—that is, child life—was growing as training and services became integrated throughout the new hospital.

Beyond the Hospital

In addition to furthering the growth of the Hopkins Child Life Program for children and families, Dombro and Haas provided a broad sense of leadership outside the hospital, reaching the local community in Baltimore as well as having an impact on psychosocial healthcare in North America.[27] They worked well with interdisciplinary teams of medical, nursing, and administrative staffs and their collaboration led to the sponsorship of several lecture series from which two books resulted. One, *The Hospitalized Child and His Family*, is a series of essays about the value of preparation, play, education, and parents living-in for hospitalized children.[28] A second book, *The Chronically Ill Child and His Family*, focused on issues of this special population.[29] They also produced a movie called *A Family Goes to the Hospital*.[30] Dombro and Haas were frequent speakers at other institutions.

One of the most noteworthy efforts of Haas's participation outside her Johns Hopkins work occurred in 1965 when she met with five other child life leaders from the United States and Canada to create the Association for the Care of Children's Health (ACCH) as a interdisciplinary organization, not just for child life. Because of her collegial work within the Hopkins Department of Pediatrics, Haas felt, as did the other women, that the way to make the greatest impact was for child life leaders to work in concert with others on the healthcare team. As a result of my serendipitous conversation with Dorothy Arnold of Goucher College, I was along for the ride. We, who were the child life instructors at Johns Hopkins, along with many play and activity leaders from around the continent, made our way to establishing an independent division within ACCH for child life specialists in the early 1970s that in time became the Child Life Council.

Eventually the child life program was transferred administratively from the nursing department at Johns Hopkins to the administration of the Johns Hopkins Children's Center. The funding shifted from the Women's Board to become a budget item in the Children's Center. Indeed, by 1967, Child Life had become a department. I was now settling in for the adventure that would come for the newly forming profession over the next 40 years.

ENDNOTES

1 Robert H. Dombro, Dan G. Kadrovach, Gerald F. Powell, and Ida Graham Price, The Child in the Hospital Environment: New Concepts of Fulfilling the Hospitalized Child's Daily Needs, *Maryland State Department of Health Monthly Bulletin, 35*(12), (1963): 1.

2 Onica Prall, Letter to Jerriann Wilson, (May 10, 1974): 1. Personal files of Jerriann Wilson.

3 Ibid., 1.

4 Ibid., 1.

5 Ibid., 2.

6 Katalin Wolff, The "Mother of Child Life" Returns to Hopkins for Visit, *The Johns Hopkins Dome, 28*(5), (1978): 8.

7 Prall, Letter to Jerriann Wilson, 2.

8 Susan R. Pincoffs, Play School, *The Johns Hopkins Nurses Alumnae Magazine, 44*(3), (July 1945): 94.

9 H. L. Mencken, Baltimore Sun Articles on The Johns Hopkins Hospital, *The Baltimore Sun*, (July 6-28, 1937): 16.

10 C. Everett Koop, Health and Health Care for the 21st Century: For All the People. *American Journal of Public Health, 96*(12), (2006): 2090.

11 Edward A. Mason, Medical Progress: The Hospitalized Child - His Emotional Needs, *The New England Journal of Medicine, 272*(8), (1965): 406-414.

12 Cindy Connolly, Growth and Development of a Specialty: The Professionalization of Child Health Care, *Pediatric Nursing, 31*(3), (2005): 213.

13 Mame Warren, *Our Shared Legacy: Nursing Education at Johns Hopkins, 1889-2006*, (Baltimore: The Johns Hopkins University Press, 2006), 51.

14 Russell A. Nelson, Memorandum to Mary S. Price, (July 7, 1961): 1.

15 J. Alex Haller, James L. Talbert, and Robert H. Dombro, eds., *The Hospitalized Child and His Family*, (Baltimore: The Johns Hopkins Press, 1967), 80.

16 Robert H. Dombro, Letter to Mary Murphy, (June 27, 1961): 1-2. Personal files of Jerriann Wilson.

17 Robert H. Dombro, Helen Schnetzer Child Life Program, *The Alumnae Magazine of the Johns Hopkins School of Nursing*, 63(1), (1964): 7-8.

18 Dombro, Helen Schnetzer Child Life Program, 8.

19 Ibid., 8.

20 Clarissa Robins Blasingame, A Comparison of the Play Material Preferences of Hospitalized and Non-Hospitalized Children, MA thesis, Purdue University, (August 1962).

21 Dombro et al., The Child in the Hospital Environment: New Concepts of Fulfilling the Hospitalized Child's Daily Needs, 3.

22 Johns Hopkins Hospital School of Nursing 1963-1964 Catalogue, (1963): 34.

23 Haller et al., *The Hospitalized Child and His Family*, 79-80.

24 Ibid., 81.

25 Ibid., 55.

26 Dombro et al., The Child in the Hospital Environment: New Concepts of Fulfilling the Hospitalized Child's Daily Needs, 84.

27 Haller et al., *The Hospitalized Child and His Family*, 86.

28 Ibid., 86.

29 Matthew Debuskey, ed., *The Chronically Ill Child and His Family*, (Springfield, IL: Charles C Thomas, 1970).

30 Haller et al., *The Hospitalized Child and His Family*, 86.

BIBLIOGRAPHY

Blasingame, Clarissa Robins. A Comparison of the Play Material Preferences of Hospitalized and Non-Hospitalized Children. MA thesis, Purdue University, August 1962.

Connolly, Cindy. Growth and Development of a Specialty: The Professionalization of Child Health Care. *Pediatric Nursing, 31*(3), (2005): 211-213, 215.

Dombro, Robert H. Letter to Mary Murphy, (June 27, 1961): 1-2.

Dombro, Robert H. Helen Schnetzer Child Life Program. *The Alumnae Magazine of the Johns Hopkins School of Nursing, 63*(1), (1964): 7-8.

Dombro, Robert H., Kadrovach, Dan G., Powell, Gerald F., & Graham Price, Ida. The Child in the Hospital Environment: New Concepts of Fulfilling the Hospitalized Child's Daily Needs. *Maryland State Department of Health Monthly Bulletin, 35*(12), (1963): 1-4.

Haller, J. Alex, Talbert, James L., & Dombro, Robert H., eds. *The Hospitalized Child and His Family*. Baltimore: The Johns Hopkins Press, 1967.

Johns Hopkins Hospital. Johns Hopkins Hospital School of Nursing 1963-1964 Catalogue, (1963).

Koop, C. Everett. Health and Health Care for the 21st Century: For All the People. *American Journal of Public Health, 96*(12) (2006): 2090-2092.

Mason, Edward A. Medical Progress: The Hospitalized Child - His Emotional Needs. *The New England Journal of Medicine, 272*(8), (1965): 406-414.

Mencken, H.L. Baltimore Sun Articles on The Johns Hopkins Hospital. *The Baltimore Sun* (July 6-28, 1937): 16.

Nelson, Russell A. Memorandum to Mary S. Price, (July 7, 1961).

Pincoffs, Susan R. Play School. *The Johns Hopkins Nurses Alumnae Magazine, 44*(3), (July 1945): 93-94.

Prall, Onica. Letter to Jerriann Wilson, (May 10, 1974).

Warren, Mame. Our Shared Legacy: Nursing Education at Johns Hopkins, 1889-2006. Baltimore: The Johns Hopkins University Press, 2006.

Wolff, Katalin. The "Mother of Child Life" Returns to Hopkins for Visit. *The Johns Hopkins Dome, 28*(5), (1978): 8.

CHAPTER 9

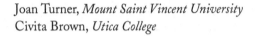

Boston Is Where It All Started: The Roots of the Child Life Study Group

Joan Turner, *Mount Saint Vincent University*
Civita Brown, *Utica College*

Mary Brooks was the first official historian for the play and activities movement that became known as the profession of child life. On May 14, 1975, she presented at the 10th Annual Conference for the Association for the Care of Children in Hospitals in order to highlight the most noteworthy milestone for the field: the first professional gathering of hospital play and education workers, titled *Patient Recreation in Pediatric Settings*.[1] As she said, it all started in Boston 1965, and on this date in 1975, the Boston tradition continued. What originated as a meeting of approximately 40 professionals from 23 hospitals had grown over a period of 10 years into a sustainable interdisciplinary organization with over 1,200 members and 1,500 conference attendees.[2] The growth in numbers only hints at the remarkable progress achieved. The vision of six founding women from play and education programs—Barbara Patterson of the Children's Hospital Medical Centre Boston; Barbara Haas (Elder) of The Johns Hopkins Hospital in Baltimore; Ruth McSweeney (Pichler) of Montreal Children's Hospital; Emma Plank of Cleveland Metropolitan General Hospital; Carol Kurtz of Pittsburgh Children's Hospital; and Mary Brooks of The Children's Hospital of Philadelphia—had been realized. Jerriann Wilson reflected on the initiative:

> They obviously had great, great wisdom because they realized that at that point, very early in 1964 and '65, that child life people by themselves couldn't really change what was happening

with children and families in hospitals all by themselves and so made the huge decision to form a multidisciplinary or interdisciplinary organization of which child life was a part. Of course, we know what happened eventually.[3]

Association for the Care of Children in Hospitals

Barbara Patterson, coordinator of patient education and recreation at the Children's Hospital Medical Center in Boston, introduced T. Berry Brazelton, M.D. to Bob Dombro of the Johns Hopkins Hospital in Baltimore and Anna Bond from Cleveland at the 1965 event.[4] Dr. Brazelton listened to each speak about their programs, and "as they talked, the artistry, the courage to fight for their aims in the face of busy hospital medicine, the obvious gains for everyone—children, families, hospital personnel, nurses, doctors (especially)—began to dawn on me. I was hooked and I have been ever since."[5]

Brazelton was the keynote speaker in Atlanta in 1973. His address not only spoke to the conference theme, "Listening to Children and their Families," but also included his perspective on the early steps in the creation of ACCH.[6] The American Association for Child Care in Hospitals (AACCH) had started out as the Association for the Well-Being of Hospitalized Children and Their Families. Brazelton noted in his keynote address his preference for the longer name, the American Association of Child and Hospital Personnel Care in Hospitals! The selection of the association name was perhaps the least difficult decision to be made during the first decade of the organization.

The first board of directors meeting was held at Brazelton's home in Cape Cod, 1967. An interim organizing committee had been formed and a transitional title chosen in 1965 followed by the establishment of a permanent organization and committee for the upcoming conference. In Baltimore, 1966, the conference title was "A Child in the Hospital Is Still a Person."[7] About 100 participants representing pediatrics, surgery, nursing, and social work, as well as the founding play and education workers, recognized the need to push forward with the formalization of the organization.[8] According to Brooks: "Those two years of organization were marked by struggle. We discussed, we argued, we even battled, as we hammered out by-laws and formulated guidelines for our developing association."[9] Ultimately, the decision to include all professions with an interest in and commitment to the care of the whole child was reached, resulting in the establishment of an

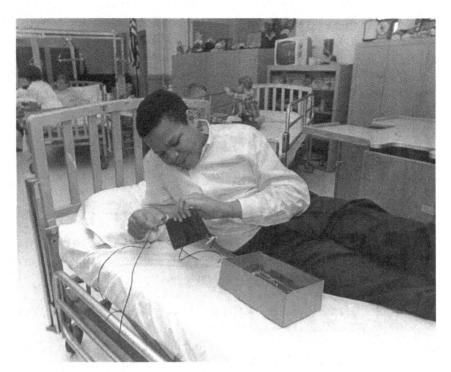

Youth with leather wallet craft in the Children's Ward at the Junior League Home

Photo courtesy of the Junior League of Nashville, Tennessee.

Reprinted by Permission from the Junior League of Nashville Tennessee.

interdisciplinary body of professionals working together to advance the interests of children in hospitals. After a long debate on whether to include pediatricians, Brazelton was especially pleased at the eventual decision to include them, "no matter how angry they may have been after such a long struggle."[10] The growth in membership over the first decade can be attributed to the interdisciplinary membership of the organization.

The achievements of such a diverse body, united in their efforts to create a forum for sharing concerns and issues around children and healthcare and to promote the growth and well-being for children in hospitals, were remarkable.[11] The Annual Conference attracted like-minded professionals across North America, and starting in 1965, annual meetings were held in Boston, Baltimore, Philadelphia, Cleveland, Ann Arbor, San Francisco, New York City, Montreal, Atlanta, and Chicago, before returning to Boston in 1975. The conference in 1967 used the name American Association for Child Care in Hospitals (AACCH); there were

225 attendees who paid a $5.00 fee for the event.[12] The first five presidents represented a striking assortment of professional disciplines, further evidence of the courage of the group to work toward a common vision. Anna Bond was a social worker directing a group program; Emma Plank came from a child development background; Helen Glaser was a pediatrician; Dean Lidgard was a special education teacher; and Carolyn Larsen Keleny had moved into a child life program from nursing. In the apt words of Mary Brooks, "It appears that the right organization was formed at the right time for the right purposes."[13]

ACCH 1965–1975

In a review of the first decade, 10 accomplishments of ACCH were presented at the conference in Boston and subsequently published in the *Journal of the Association for the Care of Children in Hospitals* that summer.[14]

1.   By 1975, the 10 affiliate ACCH groups were recognized, including Metropolitan Washington and Denver. The formation of affiliates across the country allowed more members to promote their interests in the well-being of children in hospitals to their local community.

2.   The original newsletter had advanced to the level of a professional journal by the end of 1974. Carole Klein, director of a number of child life programs in Cleveland, headed the publications committee. Conference presentations, particularly keynote addresses, were often reprinted in the publication in order to reach a broader audience. For example, Brazelton's keynote address at the 8th Annual Conference posed the question, "Can hospitalization ever be a positive experience for children?" and used the integration of research findings and practical experiences to highlight contrasting approaches. He demonstrated the potential benefits of a shift toward a strengths-based approach, viewing the stress of illness and hospitalization as an opportunity for "learning coping mechanisms and experiencing mastery over stress."[15]

Similarly, the following year, Dane Prugh, M.D. heralded the accomplishments of his friend and colleague, Sally Straub, and discussed the intertwining foundations of newly established nursery schools, hospital play and recreation, and child psychology programs at Boston Children's Hospital. One anecdote illustrating Sally's innovative approach to hospital play spoke to the changing tides affecting play and education programs across the country: "She rigged toy transfusion sets for children to play out their feelings; taught nurses how to let children in bed use play dough and red paint with covering rubber sheets, set up family-style eating arrangements, and held informal discussions with parents. Very soon her legend spread through the hospital..." [16]

3. ACCH members endeavored to write in areas of general pediatric care in their publications, which were shared worldwide. Content authors varied: pediatricians, nurses, child life professionals, and eventually parents contributed to the publication. The summer 1975 issue,[17] for example, included "Learning from Infants and Families," "Dr. Gannon and Ambulatory Care," "Centers of Learning in a Pediatric Clinic Playroom," "A Mother's Impression of Her Child's Hospitalization," "The Identification of Concerns Experienced by Fathers of Hospitalized Children," and "The Use of Guitar and Singing in a Child Life Program."

4. Pediatric parent groups were supported under the guidance of Carole Hardgrove as the parent liaison committee chair. "Living-in Accommodations and Practices for Parents in Hospital Pediatric Units," published the summer of 1975, was accompanied by articles acknowledging the perspectives of both mothers and fathers.

5. The Committee for Research was thriving. In 1974, Jacqueline Holt Vandeman, R.N., Ph.D. announced the formation of an ACCH research committee.[18] She wrote, "Dr. Cronkite...emphasized in his address here [conference 1975] the necessity for documenting of new and continuing programs. If we are to progress, research is essential in supporting our goals."[19]

6. Due to the growth of the annual conference, a planning committee was organized, and preparations for the meeting in Denver in 1976 were underway. Doris Klein's notes showed that Pat Azarnoff was the ACCH president, Carol Hardgrove was the vice-president, and B.J. Seabury was the keynote speaker, presenting on the subject of "Who Works for Children: The Realities." As recounted by Doris Klein of Children's Hospital Colorado, about one-third of the 60 conference presentations focused on play and recreation.[20]

7. Evelyn Hansbarger, previous secretary to Emma Plank in Cleveland (1970) and executive secretary for ACCH (1974), experienced new challenges: an increase in mail volume, postage to foreign countries, and the need to modernize from an eight-party line to a private telephone line. ACCH materials were mimeographed at the local church and distributed internationally. Membership as of January 19, 1974, was reported at 818 paid members.[21]

8. Concern for all children—from the youngest to the oldest—in additional healthcare settings beyond the hospital was expanding. In particular, greater attention was directed toward the unique needs of infants and adolescents. Regarding the state of child life, Carolyn Larsen of Montreal Children's Hospital, said: "[V]arious professions have been contributing to meeting commonly recognized needs, special in the pediatric milieu. In so doing, they have unwittingly parented a new and distinct professional discipline whose central aims of promoting optimal development and preventing psychological trauma in children and their families, are achieved primarily through [play...normalization...and...supportive] relationships."[22]

9. Child life and education programs were expanding. According to Mary Brooks, "Most important, many existing play programs have become more professional in nature with great emphasis on the basic needs of children, less on mere entertainment and diversion. The outdated title of 'Play Lady' will hopefully disappear as soon as we are able to find the elusive 'right title' for what is now being called Child Life/Recreation Specialist."[23] Rutkowski determined that the peak period of growth in the number of programs occurred between 1968 and 1970; likewise, individual programs were also expanding in size and scope.[24]

10. The concept of care for the whole child was advanced across hospitals and disciplines by the diligence of ACCH. Inclusion of parents in the organization membership signified a revelatory shift in pediatric attitudes. The shift away from simple diversion and entertainment of children in hospitals and towards meeting the fundamental psychosocial needs of children was beginning. New child life and education programs were emerging and had an increasing influence on the day-to-day care of children and families. Furthermore, ACCH leaders became ambassadors as they received invitations to join discussions previously exclusive to pediatricians. Emma Plank was invited to present a paper at the Annual Meeting of the American Academy of Pediatrics (AAP) and subsequently joined the committee on hospital care. Carol Hardgrove (University of California–San Francisco) was invited to participate at the International Congress of Pediatrics in Buenos Aires where hospital play was included on the agenda. Finally, a group from ACCH presented a workshop on hospital play at the Annual Meeting of the Orthopsychiatric Association.[25] ACCH appeared to be making their mark on pediatric organizations in North America.

The influence of the ACCH *parents*, aptly noted by Larsen, increased momentum for those members with roots in the play and education programs to move toward the formation of their own identity separate from the larger professional group. Although a select group of members who were beginning to self-identify as child life providers was active and engaged in the academic and scholarly activities of ACCH, there was a growing desire for more. As documented by both Rutkowski and Larsen, the expansion of child life programs signaled a need for guidance. Sally Francis recalled a group of child life specialists pondering the lack of opportunity for child life providers to "communicate among ourselves" during the interdisciplinary meetings. She noted, "We thought, wouldn't it be great if we had some separate time set aside? So we started communicating among ourselves and then lobbying within ACCH to have a child life study section."[26] By 1974, the Child Life Activity Committee was formed to help child life professionals define their identity within ACCH. In 1975, the committee title changed and became the child life activity study section (with Jerriann Wilson serving as chairperson) and for several years held pre- and postconference sessions around the ACCH Annual Conference.

Thus, the seeds of the child life profession were sown during the latter half of the 1970s. The most significant shift occurred in Dallas in 1980, following the discussion of the title of the profession at the preconference meeting on June 28. "The mercury reached 100 degrees June 7, 1980. Then it got really hot," reported The Star Telegram.[27] Jerriann Wilson and others agreed, noting "The discussion was just as hot!"[28] Those in attendance were passionate but respectful, and in the end, the group of about 60 voted unanimously (though with one abstention) in favor of the professional title of *child life*.[29]

Very soon, the roots of the early play programs would really begin to take hold during a snowstorm in Connecticut. Sally Francis captured the essence of the memorable long weekend, January 1982, stating: "Our assignment was to hammer out what we thought—between the child life specialists, the task force study section, and ACCH—would be the best way for child life specialists to move forward."[30] The ACCH-appointed leaders included Sally Francis (Texas), B.J. Seabury (Rhode Island), and Ruth Snider (Canada), all of whom joined Dr. John E. Schowalter, professor at the Yale School of Medicine Child Study Center. Sally Francis shared:

> We have just got these good vibes going on and all of a sudden
> this huge blizzard. So we had to move from the Yale Child Study

Centre and we all packed up and moved into John's [Schowalter] home. And his kids left their beds and made room for us and we sat in his living-room for two days straight looking at all of the permeations of how child life could grow. And from that, came the recommendation that there be formed a child life council. And initially the Child Life Council was under the umbrella of the Association for the Care of Children's Health and that's, we thought that would be a way to start—to have a separate council, but to still be associated under the umbrella of the Association for the Care of Children's Health. So that was a pretty significant step and I was glad to be a part of that step.[31]

Play as a Profession

The vision of the six women who were introduced at the beginning of this chapter set in motion a series of remarkable accomplishments over the period of a mere decade. That first meeting in Boston, 1965, offered a foundation for the inevitable acknowledgment of *play as a profession*: now called child life. Following that initial gathering of hospital play and recreation workers, the values of holistic care and play as a right initiated in the 1930s were moved much closer to realization for child care in hospitals. Although documentation of play initiatives goes back to the early 1900s, the "new attitude in using play" stimulated by Anne Smith and the collaborative administration at Children's Memorial Hospital Chicago eventually resulted in a growing movement.[32] While the leading ladies featured in this collection—Smith, Seabury, Brooks, and Plank—seeded their own play programs on the foundations of modern theory, the care and conditions of the pediatric milieu also modified—just not at the same pace. As noted by Carolyn Larson, "Ideally the philosophy of the hospital as a whole and that of the child life service are complementary, and there is a shared commitment to certain principles of care."[33]

History indicates that it would take the founding of the Association of the Care of Children in Hospitals and consequential interdisciplinary accomplishments to provide the conditions necessary for the complementary nature of child life services to become accepted. Indeed, perhaps it was the engagement of the hospital play and recreation workers alongside of the pediatricians, nurses, social workers, and allied healthcare providers that allowed the unique nature of child life to become articulated. For as the future will tell, consideration for the professional autonomy and authority of child life as a profession would begin to flourish—for the pips of child life had been sown in the early hospital play programs.

ENDNOTES

1 Mary McLeod Brooks, The Growth and Development of the Association for the Care of Children in Hospitals, *Journal of the Association for the Care of Children in Hospitals*, 4(1), (1975): 1-4.

2 Ibid., 2.

3 *Doris Klein: Early Days of Child Life* (video recording), (Utica, NY: Utica College, Child Life Council Archives Management Group, 2013).

4 T. Berry Brazelton, Keynote Address – 8th Annual Conference ACCH: Keeping in Touch with Children in Our Care, *Association for the Care of Children in Hospital Newsletter*, 2(2), (1974): 1-7.

5 Ibid., 1.

6 Ibid., 1.

7 Acknowledgment: Jerriann Wilson for uncovering details in her Haas-Dombro ACCH files.

8 Mary McLeod Brooks, The Growth and Development, 2.

9 Ibid., 2

10 T. Berry Brazelton, Keynote, 2.

11 Mary McLeod Brooks, The Growth and Development, 2.

12 Acknowledgment: Jerriann Wilson for uncovering details in her Haas-Dombro ACCH files.

13 Mary McLeod Brooks, The Growth and Development, 2.

14 Ibid.

15 T. Berry Brazelton, Keynote, 2.

16 Dane D. Prugh, Elizabeth M. Straub Memorial Lecture: One of the Pieces: Respect for the Cultural Heritage of the Hospitalized Child, *Journal of the Association for the Care of Children in Hospitals*, 4(2), (1975): 2.

17 Table of Contents, *Journal of the Association for the Care of Children in Hospitals*, 4(1).

18 Jacqueline Holt Vanderman, Does Research Make Any Difference in the Lives of Children? *Association for the Care of Children in Hospital Newsletter*, 2(2), (1974): 24.

19 Mary McLeod Brooks, The Growth and Development, 3.

20 *Doris Klein: Early Days of Child Life* (videorecording), (Utica, NY: Utica College, Child Life Council Archives, 2013).

21 Evelyn O. Hansbarger, Post Office Box H, *Association for the Care of Children in Hospital Newsletter*, 2(2), (1974): 9.

22 Carolyn Larsen, The Child Life Professions: Today and Tomorrow, in *Child Life an Overview* (2nd ed.), (Washington, DC: Association for the Care of Children in Hospitals, 1986), 1-10.

23 Mary McLeod Brooks, The Growth and Development, 3.

24 Jack Rutkowski, A Survey of Child Life Programs, in *Child Life an Overview* (2nd ed.), (Washington, DC: Association for the Care of Children in Hospitals, 1986), 11-15.

25 Mary McLeod Brooks, The Growth and Development, 4.

26 *CLC Yesterday, Today and Tomorrow: CLC 25th Anniversary* (DVD recording), produced and edited by Mark Santa Maria, (Utica, NY: Child Life Council Archives Management Group in partnership with Utica College and Edgewood College, 2007).

27 http://www.star-telegram.com/2010/06/06/2243599/30-years-later-north-texans-re-member.html

28 *Doris Klein: Early Days of Child Life* (videorecording), (Utica, NY: Utica College, Child Life Council Archives, 2013).

29 *Historical Overview of the Development of Child Life and the Child Life Council,* prepared by Doris Klein for the 1996 CLC Conference on Professional Issues, (Utica, NY: Child Life Council Historical Archives).

30 *CLC Yesterday, Today and Tomorrow.*

31 Ibid.

32 Clare McCausland, *An Element of Love: A History of the Children's Memorial Hospital of Chicago, Il,* (Chicago: The Children's Memorial Hospital, 1981).

33 Larson, 5.

BIBLIOGRAPHY

Brazelton, T. Berry. Keynote Address – 8th Annual Conference ACCH: Keeping in Touch with Children in Our Care. *Association for the Care of Children in Hospital Newsletter,* 2(2), (1974): 1-7.

Brooks, Mary McLeod. The Growth and Development of the Association for the Care of Children in Hospitals. *Journal of the Association for the Care of Children in Hospitals,* 4(1), (1975): 1-4.

CLC Yesterday, Today and Tomorrow: CLC 25th Anniversary (DVD recording), produced and edited by Mark Santa Maria. Utica, NY: Child Life Council Archives Management Group in partnership with Utica College and Edgewood College, 2007.

Doris Klein: Early Days of Child Life (videorecording). Utica, NY: Child Life Council Archives, 2013.

Hansbarger, Evelyn O. Post Office Box H. *Association for the Care of Children in Hospital Newsletter,* 2(2), (1974): 9.

Historical Overview of the Development of Child Life and the Child Life Council, prepared by Doris Klein for the 1996 CLC Conference on Professional Issues. Utica, NY: Child Life Council Archives.

Larsen, Carolyn. The Child Life Professions: Today and Tomorrow. In *Child Life an Overview* (2nd ed., pp. 1-10). Washington, DC: Association for the Care of Children in Hospitals, 1986.

McCausland, Clare. *An Element of Love: A History of the Children's Memorial Hospital of Chicago, Il.* Chicago: The Children's Memorial Hospital, 1981.

Prugh, Dane D. Elizabeth M. Straub Memorial Lecture: One of the Pieces: Respect for the Cultural Heritage of the Hospitalized Child. *Journal of the Association for the Care of Children in Hospitals,* 4(2), (1975): 1-8.

Rutkowski, Jack. A Survey of Child Life Programs. In *Child Life an Overview* (2nd ed., pp. 11-15). Washington, DC: Association for the Care of Children in Hospitals, 1986.

Table of Contents. *Journal of the Association for the Care of Children in Hospitals,* 4(1), (1975).

Vanderman, Jacqueline Holt. Does Research Make Any Difference in the Lives of Children? *Association for the Care of Children in Hospital Newsletter,* 2(2), (1974): 24.

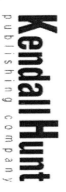

Kendall Hunt
publishing company

To PLACE an order:
Call: 800-228-0810
Fax: 800-772-9165
Mail: Kendall Hunt Cust. Service
Kendall Hunt Publishing Co.
4050 Westmark Drive
Dubuque, IA 52004-1840

To RETURN an order:
Follow the guidelines on
the Returns Policy.

Call 800-344-9031

Cust. #:	691244	Order #:	1209146-00	Order Date:	4/25/2014

B I L L T O	SYC SHARON ERIKSON INSTITUTE 451 LASALLE ST CHICAGO, IL 60654	S H I P T O	SYC SHARON CHILD LIFE PROGRAM ERIKSON INSTITUTE 451 LASALLE ST CHICAGO, IL 60654

Ship Via: UPS GD P		Ship Date:	4/28/2014	Cust. PO:	POSSIBLE ADOPT

LINE #	ITEM ISBN	TITLE AUTHOR	QUANTITY SHIPPED	UNIT PRICE	% DISCOUNT	IN BOX
1	43413901 978-1-4652-4139-9	The Pips of Child Life Turner-Brown	1	0.00	0.00	

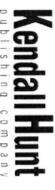

Kendall Hunt
publishing company

Kendall Hunt RETURNS Policy Effective February 1, 2010

Kendall Hunt Publishing Company always strives to ensure customer satisfaction with our products and services. Should it become necessary for you to return products, the following guidelines must be followed:

- All returned product must be carefully packaged and arrive at Kendall Hunt Publishing Company in resalable condition.
- To receive credit product must be unmarked, unstamped, un-stickered, unscratched, with no bent corners or torn covers.
- Pre-Packaged bundles must be in the original and unbroken shrink wrap.
- Software packaging seals must not be broken.

RETURNS ALLOWED: Standard and Custom Published Titles

6 months from invoice date: Bookstores, Schools, Associations, Professional Organizations, College Departments, Professors/Educators

1 month from invoice date: Individual Purchasers, Home Schools, Libraries

NO RETURNS ALLOWED:

- Digitally delivered product
- Print-on-Demand titles
- PreK-12 Book Distributors

obtained by any of the following methods:

Phone: 800-344-9031

Fax: 563-589-7032

Email: returns@kendallhunt.com <mailto:returns@kendallhunt.com>

Return instructions, including a Return Merchandise Authorization (RMA) number, will be forwarded to you upon approval. This RMA number must be placed on the exterior of each package being returned.

If the returns instructions are not followed, credit will not be issued and we will discard or return product to you at your expense.

Damaged Product: Inspect your order immediately upon arrival. If an item reaches you in damaged condition, save the shipping carton and notify Kendall Hunt at once. Do not return damaged merchandise until you receive our instructions to do so. This is necessary to facilitate a freight claim. All claims on damaged product must be made immediately upon receipt of the order (30 days or less) by contacting the Customer Service Department at 800.228.0810 or e-mail orders@kendallhunt.com

Missing or Defective Product: Call 800.228.0810 or e-mail orders@kendallhunt.com <mailto:orders@kendallhunt.com> to report any problem with your order. Be sure to thoroughly unpack your order and inspect all products, then have your packing slip or order number available when you call. Claims must be made within 30 days.

1.00

TOTAL UNITS SHIPPED: **1.00**

TOTAL # OF CARTONS: **1**

Packer ID: CLEACH